RELIGION AND MEDICAL ETHICS

The Institute of Religion Series on Religion and Health Care

The Institute of Religion was founded in 1954 by some visionaries in the Texas Medical Center who saw the importance of nurturing a conversation between medicine and religion. It was first a trailblazer in the training for hospital chaplaincy and then a trailblazer in the conversations that became the field of medical ethics.

The Institute of Religion continues to support research, education, and service at the intersection of health care and religious commitment. Books in this series are the result of theological reflection at that intersection. They are offered as a service to those in health care who want to understand and undertake their work as a calling, as a form of ministry to the sick. They are offered as a service to those in the academy who would attend — and have their students attend — to the voices of faith seeking understanding of human suffering and the responses of health care. And they are offered as a service to members of believing communities who would support, encourage, and admonish one another, including those in their midst who are sick, suffering, or dying and those in their midst with the vocation to care for the sick, suffering, or dying.

The Institute of Religion
Series on Religion and Health Care #1

Religion and Medical Ethics

Looking Back, Looking Forward

Edited by

Allen Verhey

WILLIAM B. EERDMANS PUBLISHING COMPANY
GRAND RAPIDS, MICHIGAN / CAMBRIDGE, U.K.

© 1996 Wm. B. Eerdmans Publishing Co.
255 Jefferson Ave. S.E., Grand Rapids, Michigan 49503/
P.O. Box 163, Cambridge CB3 9PU U.K.

Printed in the United States of America

01 00 99 98 97 96   7 6 5 4 3 2 1

Library of Congress Cataloging-in-Publication Data

Religion and medical ethics : looking back, looking forward /
edited by Allen Verhey.
p.   cm.
(Institute of Religion series on religion and health care : #1)
ISBN 0-8028-0862-X (alk. paper)
1. Medical ethics — Congresses.   2. Religious ethics —
Congresses.   3. Medicine — Religious aspects — Congresses.
I. Verhey, Allen. II. Series.
R725.55.R44   1996
174'.2 — dc20   96-5079
                                                  CIP

The Scripture quotations used in "Meditation" are from the Revised Standard Version of the Bible, copyrighted 1946, 1952, © 1971, 1973 by the Division of Christian Education of the National Council of Churches of Christ in the U.S.A., and used by permission.

Contents

CONTENTS

Introduction

ALLEN VERHEY

In 1968 the Institute of Religion sponsored a conference on Ethics in Medicine and Technology. It was one of the first major conferences in medical ethics in the country, and it featured religious voices. Robert Drinan, S.J., Joseph Fletcher, Paul Ramsey, and Helmut Thielicke were among those who made major addresses.

It was hardly accidental, of course, that conversations about medical ethics began in the sixties. In 1961 the technology for hemodialysis was invented, and soon choices had to be made about who was going to receive dialysis when not all those who needed it could. Questions were raised about how to make decisions that meant life to some and death to others. In the decade before Roe v. Wade (1973), abortion was already the subject of an intense national debate, and a number of states had legalized abortion. The question of when life begins, a question Roe v. Wade refused to settle, was an unavoidable part of the discussion. The first successful heart transplant, in 1967, raised the question of when life ends, the question of the definition of death. In 1966 Henry Beecher of Harvard Medical School published an article listing twenty-two medical research studies that were morally questionable. Questions were raised about using one person to obtain knowledge useful to the care of another. Developments in genetics increased human powers at the beginnings of life — for example, the ability to make prenatal diagnoses — and raised questions related to the control such powers promised over the quality of human offspring. Developments in psychiatry raised

1

questions of one person's control over the behavior or moods of another.

The new powers of medicine raised some novel moral questions in the sixties, questions beyond the considerable expertise of scientists and technicians. They were not just medical problems but moral problems, and attempts to address these questions inevitably involved some account of the significance of human life and death, of human parenting and suffering, of the goods to be sought and the limits to be imposed on seeking them.

And it was hardly accidental that religious voices were among those first responding to the questions raised by the new powers of medicine. Religious communities had long and worthy traditions of attention to the ordinary human events of giving birth and suffering and dying and of support for the extraordinary tasks of caring for those giving birth, suffering, or dying.

Daniel Callahan, one of the first and finest scholars to identify and address some of the problems posed by the new powers of medicine, acknowledged autobiographically, "When I first became interested in bioethics in the mid-1960's, the only resources were theological or those drawn from within the traditions of medicine, themselves heavily shaped by religion."[1]

Theologians and other caretakers of religious traditions played a major role in what Callahan calls "the emergence of the field"[2] and in what David Smith in this volume calls the "revival" of medical ethics. When Kenneth Vaux organized the conference on Ethics in Medicine and Technology for the Institute of Religion in 1968, it was little wonder that he called on theologians to make most of the major addresses.

The proceedings of that conference were edited by Kenneth Vaux and published under the title *Who Shall Live? Medicine, Technology, Ethics.*[3] It was an interesting and provocative book, reflecting a fascinating and productive conference. In his introduction to the book

---

1. Daniel Callahan, "Religion and the Secularization of Bioethics," *Hastings Center Report,* Special Supplement: "Theology, Religious Traditions, and Bioethics," 20, no. 4 (July–August 1990): 2.

2. Callahan, "Religion and the Secularization of Bioethics," 3.

3. Philadelphia: Fortress Press, 1970.

Kenneth Vaux called for "continuing systematic study."[4] Given the explosion of interest in and literature about medical ethics since then, that there was a time not long ago when such a call was necessary seems strange.

In 1993 the Institute of Religion sponsored a conference to celebrate the twenty-fifth anniversary of the first Houston Conference on Medicine and Technology. It was intended, of course, to remember and celebrate the first conference and the contributions of religious voices at the beginnings of bioethics, but it was not intended to be an exercise in nostalgia. Good memories have a way of pointing toward a better future. The conference looked not only back but forward: back at the contributions of theologians at the beginnings of bioethics, but also ahead to the challenges and the possibilities for speaking of bioethics with religious integrity.

In the first major paper of the conference and in the first chapter of this volume, David H. Smith, professor of religious studies and director of the Poynter Center for the Study of Ethics and American Institutions at Indiana University, looks back at the participants in the "bioethics revival." He shows not only that theologians were important to that revival but also that they entered and revived public discussion of bioethical issues precisely because of their particular religious convictions and the implications of those convictions. When at the end of his remarks he turns toward the future, he proposes a dialogue between religious and secular perspectives, a dialogue in which religious voices would neither simply provide an additional (and expendable) rationale for some generic principle nor, for the sake of preserving the richness of particular traditions, avoid such generic principles and concepts. Such a dialogue, according to Smith, has enriched and will continue to enrich both public discourse and theology.

Stephen E. Lammers, Helen H. P. Manson professor of religion at Lafayette College, looks back at "The Marginalization of Religious Voices in Medical Ethics." He points out both the reality of "marginalization" and the reasons for it, and he also shows how the process and problems of the "marginalization" of religious voices differ in different contexts, specifically in the academy, the clinic, and public

4. Kenneth Vaux, "Introduction," in *Who Shall Live? Medicine, Technology, Ethics*, xii.

policy discourse. It is a lament, in a way, but a very instructive one. It is a lament, but appreciative of the dangers when religious communities claim to speak a language that anyone and everyone should understand and accept. Indeed, he asks whether it might be appropriate not to lament but to celebrate the "marginalization" that frees religious communities to speak more critically about health care systems and professions. It is a lament, but it also points toward the hope of renewed theological engagement with medical ethics in a variety of contexts.

Two papers at the conference looked back at particular theologians who spoke at the 1968 conference and asked what may be learned from them when we turn toward the future and look ahead to the problems and possibilities of theological reflection on medical ethics. In the first of these papers, the third chapter of this volume, Karen Lebacqz, professor of Christian ethics at Pacific School of Religion, considers the work of Helmut Thielicke, one of the major contributors to the theological revival in Germany after the Second World War and one of the main speakers at the conference in 1968. She considers the concept of "alien dignity," which was so important to Thielicke, examining its theological roots and retrieving it for contemporary reflection about health care. The concept is not unproblematic, but it provides a rich legacy for the protection of human beings, for the recognition of their fundamental equality, for the acknowledgment of personal responsibility, for attention to the structural problems in health care, and for the awareness of human beings as relational. Such a legacy, according to Karen Lebacqz, can and should shape the future of theological reflection about medical ethics.

Stanley Hauerwas looks back to "the case of Paul Ramsey" in the fourth chapter. Paul Ramsey was professor of religion at Princeton University and widely acknowledged as one of the midwives at the birth or rebirth of medical ethics. He always wrote, he said, as "a Christian ethicist, and not as some hypothetical common denominator." Stanley Hauerwas, professor of theological ethics at the Divinity School, Duke University, is prepared to celebrate the candor of that statement, but he criticizes Ramsey's work for being held captive by the tradition of Protestant liberalism, by its Constantinianism, and by its confidence that the "essence" of the gospel could be articulated in terms of a transhistorical moral reality. Thus Paul Ramsey not only prepared the way for the many who followed him into reflection about medical ethics but also, ironically, prepared the way for many of those who followed him to bracket their own particular theological convictions or to ignore those of others.

It is interesting and instructive to compare this analysis and assessment of Paul Ramsey with Stephen Lammers's more general analysis of "the marginalization of religious voices." Stephen Lammers had also called attention to the "irony" of religious people turning to a language independent of their religious traditions in order to find a way to give patients a voice and then discovering, after they had succeeded, that it was difficult to speak with their own religious voice in that language. It is equally interesting and instructive to compare this account of Paul Ramsey with the proposal of David Smith concerning "paired concepts" and the effort of Karen Lebacqz to develop the notion of "alien dignity" in terms applicable to contemporary issues in health care ethics. These are proposals and models for the relation of religious ethics to other sources of moral insight that are important for the future of theological reflection about the ethics of health care.

That relation is the direct focus of the analytical piece by James M. Gustafson, "Styles of Religious Reflection in Medical Ethics." Professor Gustafson was himself one of the people who began to comment on issues of morality in health care long before there was a discernible field of inquiry called "bioethics." He was one of the first theologians to lament the fact that when people with theological training commented on issues of medicine and technology, they seldom called on their religious traditions or theological convictions.[5] He remains one of the most astute observers of the practices and problems of moral theologians as they consider contemporary moral issues and turn toward the future. His sketch of three "ideal-types," the autonomy of religious ethics, the intelligibility of religious ethics, and the dialectic of religious ethics, provides a heuristic device for examining the strengths and weaknesses of ways of working within religious traditions in conversation with others about medical ethics. As he observes, the force of his analysis is not to constrain a selection of one way of working; different

5. See James M. Gustafson, "Theology Confronts Technology and the Life Sciences," *Commonweal*, 16 June 1978, 386-92.

strategies may be appropriate to different occasions and audiences; however, this heuristic device enables those who engage in theological reflection about health care to be more self-conscious and more self-critical of the strategies they adopt to articulate their religious tradition in public (and pluralistic) places.

The last major address of the conference, and chapter six of this book, looks forward to the future by identifying a facet of the moral life too much neglected in conventional bioethics, a feature of the moral life that religious traditions are well suited to nurture and sustain. Warren T. Reich is professor of bioethics and director of health and humanities at Georgetown University; he served as editor-in-chief of the *Encyclopedia of Bioethics* and of its current revision. His account of "A New Era for Bioethics: The Search for Meaning in Moral Experience" sets an agenda for religious communities and their theologians that would focus less on dilemmas and more on character, less on decisions about actions and more on attentiveness to the suffering, less on preserving the autonomy of strangers and more on the disposition and the wisdom to care for embodied and communal people whose sickness threatens to alienate them from their communities, from those who would care for them, and from themselves. It suggests the possibility and the necessity of another "revival" in medical ethics and the possibility and the necessity of religious voices leading the way toward such a future.

An important part of the conference, in addition to the six papers provided in the first six chapters of this book, was the working groups. Reports of their reflections and conclusions are provided in chapters seven and eight. One set of working groups considered various contexts for medical ethics, the academy, the medical center, the religious community, and the law or public policy. Each working group looked back a little at the role of religious voices in their particular context, but they also looked ahead to the challenges and possibilities for those who wanted to work with religious integrity within that context. The results of their conversations were reported to the group and are summarized in chapter seven. A second set of working groups focused on particular issues — abortion, genetics, assisted suicide, and access to health care. Again each group looked back a little, making some summary and assessment of theological reflection about this issue in the past, and again each working group attempted to look forward, identifying elements of an agenda for theological reflection about this particular issue. The results of their work are summarized in chapter eight.

The conference also included a worship service. It was appropriate to give thanks to God, to acknowledge the limits of our medicine and of our medical ethics, and to be attentive for a little while to the One to whom we would be attentive all the while. The worship service, including its meditation, is also included in this volume.

The publication of these papers is undertaken in the confident hope that they will nurture and inform theological reflection in various contexts and about diverse issues. It is also undertaken in grateful remembrance of the stewardship that has sustained the vision of the founders of the Institute of Religion, the vision of conversation and cooperation between health care and religious communities.

Special thanks are due to the people who helped make the conference and these proceedings possible. The Memorial Drive Presbyterian Church provided a grant for the conference. Dr. Jan van Eys made a personal contribution and supported the conference from the beginning as the president of the board of trustees of the Institute of Religion. Kenneth Vaux, who organized the first conference, was very helpful. Jon Pott, of Eerdmans Publishing Company, provided valuable advice from the beginning of the project. Those who participated in the conference and in the working group made it a delightful as well as an instructive occasion. The staff of the Institute of Religion worked hard to make the event seem effortless.

Religion and the Roots
of the Bioethics Revival

DAVID H. SMITH

I want to offer a diagnosis and prescription for the role of religion in the bioethics discussion in the United States. I begin with a short history, turn to a brief comment about the present state of affairs, and conclude with a recommendation. I speak as one eager to see religious ideas used — in the best sense of the word, *exploited* — in the bioethics discussion. I believe that the absence of religious perspectives and ideas greatly impoverishes that discussion.

Was religion present at the creation? Thirty years ago a bioethics revival began. Who started and shaped it? In identifying the players at the outset of the bioethics revival, I make no claim for comprehensiveness. Different persons would surely make somewhat different lists, and mine is not without its problems; I risk some sweeping generalizations. I omit the many physicians who played a crucial role in the revival of interest in medical ethics, because I want to focus on the nonmedical response to the new powers and problems of medicine, to check the thesis that religious thought was important to the revival, and not just accidentally. The religious character of the perspective of many scholars led to their entering and reviving the public discussions of issues in bioethics.

One important set of players at the outset comprised some maverick philosophers; they were scholars whose intellectual odyssey had put them somewhere outside the mainstream of establishment

9

academic philosophy, but they nevertheless were clearly identifiable as philosophers. Some of these persons knew religious thought and theological ethics. This group included, for example, Daniel Callahan, who had written on issues of the sort we now call practical ethics, had served as the editor of *Commonweal,* and had set to work on his book on abortion.[1] Callahan's identity as a Catholic was then very clear, whatever disagreements he may have had with the hierarchy or with existing Catholic moral theology. The bioethics revival, after all, roughly coincided with the Second Vatican Council. It is hard to imagine what the bioethics revival would have been like without the Hastings Center, shaped as it largely has been by Callahan's philosophical perspective — a perspective that is still recognizably Catholic, however Callahan's loyalties or engagements may have changed.

Another thinker whose work is best described under this heading was Hans Jonas, whose early essay on experimentation with human subjects[2] was to prove to be extraordinarily influential. Before his work in bioethics, Jonas was best known in this country for his interpretative study *The Gnostic Religion,*[3] done while he was in Germany and clearly influenced by the thought of Heidegger and Bultmann. That work may lie far in the background of Jonas's work in biomedical ethics, but at a minimum it signaled Jonas's religious and theological literacy and concerns. Indeed, religious texts and concerns came somewhat more to the fore in his later writings; for example, Jonas was mightily concerned with suffering, with insights about suffering that could be found in religious images or traditions; he realized that theological formulations captured some aspects of suffering — notably the fact that persons can grow through suffering — that many nonreligious intellectual formulations leave out of account.

A second very important player was one of a kind. Joseph Fletcher, then clearly seeing himself as an Episcopal priest, had written *Morals and Medicine,*[4] which antedated the bioethics revival by a decade. Fletcher's career before *Morals and Medicine* had included leadership in various

---

1. Daniel Callahan, *Abortion: Law, Choice, and Morality* (New York: Macmillan, 1970).

2. Hans Jonas, "Philosophical Reflections on Experimenting with Human Subjects," *Daedalus* 98, no. 2 (Spring 1969): 219-47.

3. Hans Jonas, *The Gnostic Religion* (Boston: Beacon Press, 1963).

4. Joseph Fletcher, *Morals and Medicine* (Boston: Beacon Press, 1960).

Episcopal social action movements and the editing of a helpful little book called *Christianity and Property*.[5] *Morals and Medicine* advanced strong arguments about truth telling and care for the dying. It concluded with one of the most persuasive statements of his ethics that Fletcher ever offered: a focus on personalism and the rights of individuals.

A third set of players who served as midwives to the rebirth of bioethics included Helmut Thielicke,[6] Karl Barth,[7] Dietrich Bonhoeffer,[8] and other Protestant writers associated with what is often called neoorthodoxy. The neoorthodox movement was close to the apogee of its influence in the intellectual world of Protestant theology as the bioethics revival began. Thielicke's *The Ethics of Sex* was widely used and portions were heavily anthologized. The long discussions of euthanasia and abortion — not to mention the sections on creation, covenant, and human relations — in III/4 of Barth's *Church Dogmatics* were widely read in seminaries and graduate programs.

Fourth, although H. Richard Niebuhr had been dead for several years, his influence in theological ethics continued to grow, and was clearly visible in the writings of several of the first wave of writers in bioethics. We can identify two different trajectories. The clearest line is from Niebuhr to the work of James M. Gustafson. Although Gustafson's views have changed — at least in emphasis[9] — he has always stressed God's transcendence of all human purposes. This has led to great sensitivity to the complexity of the challenges facing selves seeking to trust in and be loyal to God. The results of this trajectory have been appreciation for ambiguity and great sensitivity to particularity and the importance of balancing competing interests.

A somewhat different line may be traced from the metaphor of

5. Joseph Fletcher, ed., *Christianity and Property* (Philadelphia: Westminster Press, 1947).

6. Helmut Thielicke, *The Ethics of Sex,* trans. John W. Doberstein (New York: Harper & Row, 1964).

7. Karl Barth, *Church Dogmatics III/4: The Doctrine of Creation,* trans. A. T. Mackay et al. (Edinburgh: T. & T. Clark, 1961).

8. Dietrich Bonhoeffer, *Ethics,* trans. Neville Horton Smith (New York: Macmillan, 1955).

9. Compare the tone of James M. Gustafson, *Christ and the Moral Life* (New York: Harper & Row, 1968), with *Ethics from a Theocentric Perspective* (Chicago: University of Chicago Press, 1981).

covenant, a leitmotif in Niebuhr's constructive work,[10] to the application of this metaphor in diverse ways to questions of medical ethics. The idea is dominant in the work of Paul Ramsey; it was central in his *Basic Christian Ethics*[11] and served as the foundation for *The Patient as Person.*[12] Ramsey's controlling idea was that the relation between physician and patient should be a covenantal one; that meant for him partnership — recognition of the patient as a self — and common commitment to purpose on the part of patient and physician. William F. May has also developed the covenantal theme, if in a different style. It is present in his earliest essays in the field and, of course, in his book *The Physician's Covenant.*[13]

Fifth, Catholic moral theology was a player at the revival of medical ethics — and present in abundance. For Bernard Häring,[14] Richard McCormick, S.J.,[15] and Charles Curran,[16] many of the issues had been part and parcel of their training. The debate over *Humanae Vitae,* the papal encyclical on contraception, heated the discussion, and they were concerned to reformulate Catholic moral theology and then to apply these reformulations to the great issues of bioethics — new bottles for wine that was new, but recognizably wine. For Germain Grisez[17] and John Finnis,[18] the wine wasn't new, but the formulations and distinctions were original and powerful.

10. See, for example, H. Richard Niebuhr, "The Idea of Covenant and American Democracy," *Church History* 23, no. 2 (June 1954): 126-35.

11. Paul Ramsey, *Basic Christian Ethics* (New York: Charles Scribner's Sons, 1950).

12. Paul Ramsey, *The Patient as Person* (New Haven: Yale University Press, 1970).

13. William F. May, *The Physician's Covenant: Images of the Healer in Medical Ethics* (Philadelphia: Westminster Press, 1983).

14. Bernard Häring, *Medical Ethics* (Notre Dame: Fides Publishers, 1973).

15. Richard McCormick, S.J., *How Brave a New World?* (New York: Doubleday and Company, 1981).

16. Charles E. Curran, *Contemporary Problems in Moral Theology* (Notre Dame: Fides Publishers, 1970).

17. Germain Grisez, *Abortion: The Myths, the Realities, and the Arguments* (New York: Corpus Books, 1970).

18. John M. Finnis, "Three Schemes of Regulation," in John T. Noonan, Jr., ed., *The Morality of Abortion: Legal and Historical Perspectives* (Cambridge: Harvard University Press, 1970).

Finally, traditional Judaism was a player. Fred Rosner,[19] David Feldman,[20] Immanuel Jakobovits,[21] and David Bleich[22] had a distinctive perspective on these issues, and they were certainly not caught unprepared by the new intellectual movement.

It would not be hard to extend this list. For example, the great sociologist Renee C. Fox, who has always been sensitive to the role of religious metaphors and experience, could be added to the list.[23] But the points are, I trust, obvious: religion was present at the creation of bioethics as we know it today, and the religious interest in and influence upon the revival of medical ethics can be (and must be) traced to the intrinsic force of the religious ideas held by these players.

To reinforce the point, consider: who was absent? The list above is pretty extensive, but it does exclude some parties. For example, mainline philosophy was not, to start with, a serious player. It is wrong, I think, to imagine academic moral or social philosophy in the sixties as unconcerned with normative questions, but it was not particularly concerned with questions of bioethics — nor is it today, any more than mainline departments of religious studies are. Still, there has been a real change in philosophy. It should not surprise or shock us that philosophy, as an academic field, was slow to get engaged. Religious ethics has historically been related to the church, synagogue, or other religious community — to the behavior and choices facing real people and groups. In contrast, academic philosophy has had no comparable responsibility or engagement with nonacademic contexts and has shared the twentieth-century academy's preoccupation with method, with theoretical clarity and elegance. In this respect religious studies, at the end of the century, is more like philosophy than religious scholarship was in an earlier generation.

Scholars whose main intellectual formation in religion or theol-

---

19. Fred Rosner, *Modern Medicine and Jewish Law* (New York: Yeshiva University Department of Special Publications, 1972).

20. David Feldman, *Marital Relations, Birth Control, and Abortion in Jewish Law* (New York: Schocken Books, 1974).

21. Immanuel Jakobovits, *Jewish Medical Ethics* (New York: Bloch, 1959).

22. J. David Bleich, *Contemporary Halakhic Problems* (New York: KTAV, 1977).

23. Renee C. Fox, *The Courage to Fail: A Social View of Organ Transplants and Dialysis* (Chicago: University of Chicago Press, 1974); *Experiment Perilous: Physicians and Patients Facing the Unknown* (Glencoe, Ill.: Free Press, 1959).

ogy lay in the thought of Reinhold Niebuhr — whether they taught in colleges, universities, or seminaries — also were not especially concerned with bioethics. For them the most important issues were those of justice within and among nations: questions of civil rights, economic injustice, and war. The topics of bioethics seemed to them to be matters of scrupulosity, appropriate subjects only of private judgment. The really interesting moral issues lay elsewhere.

Moreover, the Bultmannians and other Continental theologians of the left, that is, the protoliberationists and the real liberationists, although they differed with the political thought of Reinhold Niebuhr and his followers, nevertheless agreed with them that the real issues were social and political in another sense. Many of the questions that concerned the first wave of work in bioethics, for example, concern with the definition of death, in vitro fertilization, and euthanasia, must have seemed to them to be simply obfuscation of the real issues of political and economic hegemony. This is not to deny the great preoccupation with professional power and dominance among many of the first and still leading writers in the bioethics field.

My impression is that the Niebuhrian and liberation theologies tend to be most at home in seminaries, whereas concern with bioethics has been concentrated in religion departments in colleges and universities. Part (but only part) of the reason for this lies in the tendency of seminaries to take a prophetic role vis-à-vis the church, to interpret their task as helping religious persons break out of self-absorption and into concern with the larger world. At any rate, the unfortunate corollary has been to lay a seminaries-versus-religious-studies grid on top of the bioethics-versus-political-ethics grid. One sad consequence of this is that Christian bioethics has not been as sensitive to the social character of selfhood as it might be; another is that much too little work on bioethics has been done in seminaries.

On my reading that was the landscape in religious and moral thought in which bioethics emerged. What has happened since then? I will be brief here because this is the subject of Stephen Lammers's essay, but I want to make a couple of observations because they are relevant to my effort to make a suggestion for future religious work in bioethics.

First, although Fletcher did very little formal training of students and was not really an academic writer, the very American stress on personal autonomy that concludes *Morals and Medicine* has been highly influential, perhaps the dominant strand in bioethics, even religiously rooted bioethics. It is a central theme in the work of Robert Veatch[24] and James Childress,[25] leading scholars in bioethics and both more academic and nuanced writers than Fletcher.

Second, the changed role of religion or theology in bioethics — if such in fact there be — is not especially a function of changed attitudes toward religion, certainly not increased hostility toward religion, in departments of philosophy, across the academy, or in the culture generally. My experience is that scholars and practitioners *outside religious or theological faculties* are actually very interested in the normative import or insight associated with relevant religious terms, concepts, and perspectives — more interested, for example, than the historians within religious studies. To be sure, they resist being treated as if they believe something they do not — but who can blame them for that?

The fact is that religiously informed thinkers were so influential at the beginning of the bioethics movement because a standpoint within a religious tradition helped them to say things that were true and insightful. Ramsey's idea that experimenters and their subjects should be seen as partners,[26] Gustafson's insistence that a traditional way of analyzing the abortion question ignored crucial variables, that it wasn't so much wrong as incomplete[27] — these points were not persuasive *because* they were religious; they were persuasive because they got at something clearly right. The religious traditions, or communities of discourse, or spokespersons were listened to precisely because it was obvious that they had something important to say. Religion was associated with a fund of insight into human relations and destiny, and the traditions could be drawn on and reinterpreted to great effect.

If we then ask, what has happened to religion in the bioethics discussion, my inclination is to say that it is still very much around.

24. Robert M. Veatch, *A Theory of Medical Ethics* (New York: Basic Books, 1981).

25. James F. Childress, *Who Should Decide? Paternalism in Health Care* (New York: Oxford University Press, 1982).

26. Ramsey, *Patient as Person*, 1-58.

27. James M. Gustafson, "A Protestant Ethical Approach," in Noonan, ed., *Morality*, 101-22.

DAVID H. SMITH

Thank God, several of the figures to whom I have referred in the present perfect tense are still working at top form; among my contemporaries a respectable fraction of the leading scholars in bioethics operate from a religiously informed sensibility, and for some — including many of those present at this conference — the religious concepts, traditions, and distinctions are high profile. What has been lacking in my generation, I think, is the sustenance of a theological perspective that allows someone to move into the public arena as Ramsey or Gustafson or May or Thielicke or McCormick has done. We have tended either to push theology into the background, making it simply a rationale for autonomy and justice (or the troubling excesses of beneficence), or to preserve richness of insight at the cost of forsaking conversation with the world.

In conclusion then, and as part of an effort to look ahead, I will suggest one way this intellectual perspective might be sustained and nurtured. I will call it the paired concepts proposal. My extremely rough idea is that we might be able to single out some key terms in public debate that roughly correlate with others that have retained more theological substance. Then members of religious communities could and should defend the "secular" concept, use it to criticize the theological one, and push it in a direction that coheres with the theological one. Let me give three quick examples.

The archetypal case for my proposal is Reinhold Niebuhr's love-justice dialectic.[28] Niebuhr thought that love was the core Christian moral norm; it was dialectically related to equality, which he once called "love in terms of logic." All sorts of problems came up, he thought, if one recommended love as a relevant social standard. For example, loving people may submit to injustice when they should not. But Niebuhr did not conclude that the norm of love was irrelevant or unnecessary. Love was a necessary and helpful corrective. Love provided a reason for defending equality; its excesses could be constrained by equality; it suggested a characteristic interpretation of equality.

If we applied this dialectic to the debate over the provision of health care — especially if we situated it within Niebuhr's larger vision

28. See Harry R. David and Robert C. Good, eds., *Reinhold Niebuhr on Politics* (New York: Charles Scribner's Sons, 1960).

16

— the effect would be to be concerned with equality of access but also to seek pragmatic solutions and compromises rather than sentimental compassion or ideological purity, that is, insistence on absolute equality or nothing. What counts is that those who are not now getting care get it. We must push the structures of power toward a more equitable access. We will never get to loving care for all; we better be sure we more closely approximate equality than we now do.

We see another pairing or dialogue in William F. May's discussion of the concepts of covenant and contract as alternative norms for the relationship between physician and patient.[29] Covenant is the clearly religious term, central in Judaism and Christianity. It is an ideal standard for professional relations; contract is but a partial translation of covenant language into the moral idiom of the day. Contract language leads to excessive concern with issues of power; it can go hand in hand with a minimalist conception of one's role. Thus, seeing oneself as contracted is finally inadequate for a professional. But contract language does represent a real advance on an ethic of status relations; moreover, it safeguards the professional against the excessive demands and the paternalism that seeing oneself in the role of a covenant partner can produce.

Let me offer one more example, this one of my own design and much more tentative. One issue that troubles much of the medical ethics discussion is the question of goals. If we want to set limits, if we want to provide access, if we want to establish norms for a professional relationship, the question of goals inevitably comes up. What is the end or objective of medicine? Several contenders for this honor are at play. Sometimes the idea seems to be to "maximize human freedom"; sometimes it is to maximize happiness or minimize pain; in some of the genetics literature it seems to be to direct evolution toward some particular vision of ideal humanity, or at least away from a clearly identifiable list of human ills.

Against these possibilities — and as a radical alternative to some of them — Christians might think of the *transfigured self,* by which I mean a self perfected through acceptance of limit, suffering, and service. It is the self of discipleship, in Christian theological terms.

---

29. William F. May, *The Physician's Covenant: Images of the Healer in Medical Ethics* (Philadelphia: Westminster Press, 1983).

That, not a life of maximized freedom or happiness, is the ideal life — although Christians will claim it brings freedom and happiness in train.

I do not think the idea of the transfigured self will play in Peoria — or in the medical center in Peoria — but I do think we can talk about human *dignity,* affirm freedom's importance to it, and then go on to argue for some other components of respect and dignity that relate clearly to the more theological concept. For example, dignity is not found without commitment or simply in maximizing pleasure. On the other hand, stressing human dignity gives us purchase against theological schools or movements that make suffering or imperfections ends in themselves, that ignore the importance of liberation from bondage to convention, or that deny the joy associated with the hope of the resurrection that follows crucifixion.

These ideas are obviously embryonic; the proposal itself needs development; an advantage is that nurturing these ideas and this proposal would invite a dialogue between secular and religious perspectives. Whatever the merits of the proposal, I remain convinced that the religious influence at the beginnings of bioethics was strong, that it arose from the intrinsic force of the ideas offered by religious writers, and that it has waned much less than one might suppose. The report of its demise can be greatly exaggerated.

We should look for fruitful ways publicly to express the insights found in religious traditions. This may or may not mean translation from one set of concepts into another; it may mean reinterpreting concepts with an eye to their contemporary relevance. The dialogue that results may enrich theology as well as the public conversation.

The Marginalization
of Religious Voices in Bioethics

STEPHEN E. LAMMERS

Introduction

It is a pleasure to be invited to be a small part of the anniversary celebration of the conference on ethics in medicine sponsored by the Institute of Religion twenty-five years ago. In his letter of invitation, Allen Verhey asked me to reflect on the reasons why religious voices were marginalized, and whether it is good for public discourse in bioethics for religious voices to be muted. What was not clear from the letter of invitation was *for whom* the religious voices were marginalized. That point is important because my own work in bioethics takes place in the clinic and in the academy. The world of physicians and nurses might turn out to be very different from the world of those of us who work primarily in the academy. Further, it may be different from the world(s) inhabited by the undergraduates whom we teach. I hope to show in what follows that there is no single or simple answer to the question of marginalization, given the different audiences in our society today.

Before going any further, let me offer a working description of marginalization. For purposes of this paper, marginalization refers to the lack of a public voice for persons with religious convictions. The issue emphatically is not whether religious voices dominate or do not dominate discussions in bioethics; the issue is whether religious voices are recognized as potential partners within public conversations —

that is, within the conversations to which we are all invited[1] — or are deemed to be relevant only in those private conversations that are encouraged to flourish, but flourish apart from the public conversations of our society.

Background to the Discussion

The topic of the marginalization of religious voices, or variants of it, has been very popular of late. Indeed, it is almost a growth industry. What has been claimed is that bioethics, as it has developed in the United States, has effectively excluded religious voices as the field of bioethics has developed. There seems to be some evidence for this claim. As just one piece of evidence for the claim that religious voices were once a part of the conversation of bioethics, but now are not, we can recall the National Commission for the Protection of Human Subjects, which produced *The Belmont Report* and other documents concerning experimentation on human subjects. If we compare that work to a recently funded federal grant on educating health care ethics committees, what do we find? For the National Commission, although the theologians' remarks did not appear in the various reports, at least theologians were asked to produce papers for that body and theologians spoke on how and why human subjects ought to be protected. Although theological language was not used in the final documents, theologians were discussion partners.[2] It may well be that the National Commission was a turning point in this matter, but that would be another discussion.[3]

1. Whether these public conversations are the important conversations within society is another matter entirely.
2. Cf. Stanley Hauerwas, "Rights, Duties and Experimentation on Children: A Critical Response to Worsfold and Bartholome," in *Appendix to Report and Recommendations, Research Involving Children* (Washington, D.C.: Superintendent of Documents, 1977); Richard A. McCormick, S.J., "Experimentation on the Fetus: Policy Proposals," and Paul Ramsey, "Moral Issues in Fetal Research," in *Appendix: Research on the Fetus* (Washington, D.C.: Superintendent of Documents, 1976).
3. On the language of the National Commission for the Protection of Human Subjects, see the first footnote in Karen Lebacqz, "Humility in Health Care," *The Journal of Medicine and Philosophy* 17 (1992): 291-307.

The Belmont Report was issued in 1979. In the more recent case of the syllabus on educating health care ethics committees, issued in 1993, not only is there no place in the curriculum for theological perspectives, there is also no place in the curriculum for a discussion of different religions, how those different religions might approach all or parts of the current health care system, or how different religions might have special perspectives on disputed matters within bioethics. Clearly something has changed.[4]

The evidence of marginalization can be followed through by looking at who are the major speakers at conferences, the themes at these conferences, and the agenda of bioethics. Very few of the conferences on bioethics, unless organized under religious auspices, attend to religious voices. The only caveat here is that conferences that take seriously the pluralism of our culture do attend to different religious perspectives, although when that happens, most often religions are simply objects of study and not systems of thoughtfulness from which we might learn something. Religious voices are thus a curiosity and not something to be taken seriously, except insofar as one might need to know about a particular religion in order to treat patients.

But it should be noted that it is not only religious voices that have been muted or marginalized in mainline bioethics. Our colleagues who are interested in feminist studies would point out that traditional accounts of medical ethics were male centered and male dominated. It was not simply that women's voices were not present; women's experience was devalued. Feminist and religious voices have in common a worry about the dominant voice in bioethics. This does not mean that they are united in what they think ought to be done about it.[5]

Earlier, I claimed that the topic of the marginalization of reli-

---

4. Cf. Stuart F. Spicker and Judith Wilson Ross, "Grant Proposal for the Fund for the Improvement of Postsecondary Education: Educating Healthcare Ethics Committees," *HEC Forum* 5, no. 1 (1993): 52-71.

5. An interesting paper could be written comparing and contrasting feminist reactions to this marginalization of women to some of the theological community's responses to the marginalization of religious voices. I do not assume for a moment that those categories are exclusive.

On feminist bioethics, cf. Helen Bequaert Holmes and Laura M. Purdy, eds., *Feminist Perspectives in Medical Ethics* (Bloomington, Ind.: Indiana University Press, 1992).

gious voices in bioethics sometimes reminds me of a small growth industry. It is, however, a growth industry only in certain circles; the question assumes a particular social location, namely, the academy and those institutions associated with the academy. This topic is relevant primarily to those persons who have adopted what Linnell Cady and others have called the Enlightenment understanding of reason, in which judgments are based on empirical evidence and are potentially confirmable by all persons who can reason.[6] In that world, religious voices have been marginalized; and for persons who wish to live in that world and at the same time to think theologically, there is a problem. Insofar as medicine is part of the academy, there has been a marginalization of religious voices there as well, at least in the published work in bioethics that appears in medical journals. I will spend some time pointing out how I think this marginalization has affected the medical profession, for I do think that the effects there are different than in the academy. For example, there has not been a response there to this marginalization, such as has developed among certain theologians within the academy. A third realm of discourse in which religious voices have been marginalized, as I noted above, is in the public policy discussions that are part and parcel of bioethics in our society.

In a helpful essay on this topic, Martin Marty takes the muting of religious voices as a given and argues that there are a number of factors that account for how this occurred. He points to long-term trends in our society toward differentiation of tasks, so that the religious and spiritual realms of existence are separated from the scientific and the political. This has happened not only at the level of ideas but at the level of institutions. One has only to consider all of the educational and medical functions that were once the exclusive domain of the churches and that are now performed by many different institutions, including the state itself. But Marty goes on suggestively to state that this is not simply a matter of one institution picking up the function of another institution. The Enlightenment project had its effects within religious communities as well. For example, the status of the theologian in religious communities them-

6. Linnell E. Cady, *Religion, Theology, and American Public Life* (Albany, N.Y.: State University of New York Press, 1993), 35ff.

selves has become ambiguous, as the theologian participates in the life of the secular university. The result is to render problematic the theologian's authority in speaking for the community, as well as the role of the theologian within the community, speaking to the community. Marty adds that in addition to the above factors, some religious thinkers desire a basis for morality that transcends any particular religious beliefs. Pluralism, secularization, and the yearnings of Western academic theologians to participate in the ethos of the academy have all contributed to the marginalization of religious voices. Moreover, as Marty points out, in this process religious people often have been active participants as well as unwilling bystanders.[7]

Marty argues further that if one reflects on the circumstances under which bioethics began to enter into the clinical realm, one notices that there was a desire to find some way of giving patients a voice in the face of powerful medical technologies and the keepers of those technologies. The language that was used, it was thought, should be a language that anyone could use. A language dependent on one religious tradition did not seem open enough for these purposes. The consequence was, of course, that there appeared to be no room for religious voices. This was a result, not a goal, of the introduction of bioethics into the clinic, an introduction often aided and abetted by religious people in their desire to assist patients in regaining a voice. Thus, in one of those ironies that mark the human condition, we find religious people helping hospitals form ethics committees and bringing bioethics issues to the attention of the medical and nursing staff. What these same religious people did not realize was that the language they were often using would minimize, undercut, or downplay the significance of their own religious commitments.

Now neither Marty nor this author is suggesting that there was once a "golden age" in which religious voices were somehow normative in bioethical discussion. But if Marty is correct, and he certainly does not stand alone here, something has happened that calls for reflection. What I would like to do now is to turn to the different settings of bioethics in our society: first, the academy; second, what I shall call

7. Martin Marty, "Religion, Theology, Church, and Bioethics," *The Journal of Medicine and Philosophy* 17 (1992): 273-89.

medicine and the clinic; and third, public policy discussions. I will end with some tentative conclusions. I hope to show that the marginalization of religious voices has affected each of these three groups slightly differently, and I hope to provide a framework that will enable us to carry on a more nuanced conversation about this topic.

The Academy

It is not surprising that religious voices have been muted within the academy. If we are candid on this point, we must admit that religious voices are often suspect within the academy. The modern university is an offspring of the Enlightenment, and the Enlightenment arose as an attempt to overcome the kinds of fractious and lethal religious division that led to events such as the Hundred Years' War and the continuing forms of religious division that are lethal even in our own day. As opposed to the particularity of religious voices, we are told that we should strive for some universal understanding that permits all persons to make arguments for their conception of a good life and that, furthermore, we should seek political and social arrangements that do not permit anyone to impose their conception of a good life upon others. When this is worked out for bioethics, the standard account claims that it is better that persons learn the basic principles of beneficence, autonomy, nonmaleficence, and justice, and apply them to the issues at hand. There is no need for the language(s) of a particular religion. If religious voices were permitted into bioethics, the fear is, we would be subject to the kind of fractious religious division that marks some of the public discussions of abortion in this country. Better that religious visions and religious voices be kept from bioethics. Not so incidentally, the recommendations from the academy for medicine and the clinic are clear. Patients should be permitted their visions of a good life, and what physicians and nurses should learn to do is to respect the patients without making any assessments of the patients' plans for a good life.

There is much to be said for this approach. First, the desire for a form of moral discourse that would be plausible across religious boundaries is not solely an Enlightenment ideal. Some religious people have shared that goal. Second, attention to the four

24

principles of nonmaleficence, beneficence, justice, and respect for persons presumably would give us standards for moral critique and moral justification. In a pluralistic society, fragmented as ours is, as Courtney Campbell reminds us, this would be no small accomplishment.[8]

This accomplishment does not come without costs. The focus is on procedure. This is not a substantive position that claims that it is grounded in some vision of who we are and where we are going. All it promises us is a way of proceeding in a society so culturally diverse as our own. But again, this is no small feat.

However, this standard account is not without its critics in the academy. Let me see if I can capture one compelling critique of the bioethics about which I am speaking. This particular critique runs as follows: The difficulty with the standard bioethics is that it is the bioethics of the person from anywhere (or from nowhere). It pretends to a universality that it does not deserve; it does not reflect on the fact that it too has a history, that it has developed as a part of and in reaction to certain historical factors, and thus it is particular — indeed, just as particular as any religious vision. The pretension to universality and neutrality, and all that accompanies it, must be punctured.[9]

Some critics who are speaking out of religious traditions go on to suggest that there are reasons for religious thinkers to reject the philosophical worldview underlying this standard form of bioethics. This worldview teaches us that we are the authors of our lives, in brief, that we are gods. But this is precisely what these thinkers argue is false to their own religious views.[10]

Other critics take a different approach. They argue that the standard bioethics is inadequate as a full account of the moral life, and

8. Courtney S. Campbell, "Principlism and Religion: The Law and the Prophets," in Edwin R. DuBose, Ronald P. Hamel, and Laurence J. O'Connell, eds., *A Matter of Principles: Ferment in U.S. Bioethics* (Valley Forge, Pa.: Trinity Press International, 1994), 183-212.

9. The standard work here is Alasdair MacIntyre, *After Virtue,* 2nd ed. (Notre Dame: University of Notre Dame Press, 1984).

10. Cf. Stanley Hauerwas, "Salvation and Health: Why Medicine Needs the Church," in *Suffering Presence* (Notre Dame: University of Notre Dame Press, 1986), 63-83.

too often it fails to recognize its own limitations. When it is taken as sufficient, it turns out to be perverse. If it were to recognize its limitations, all could be well.[11]

Thus within the academy, what we find is a marginalization of religious voices, but a countermovement as well. Not only has the marginalization been noticed, but critique and countercritique are the order of the day. The debates appear in some journals that are mainstays of bioethics as well as in the academic philosophical literature. Thus there have been symposia not only in *The Journal of Philosophy and Medicine,*[12] but also in *The Hastings Center Report.*[13] What is mixed is the evidence about whether these symposia have made any impact on the way bioethics is taught outside the university, especially in the medical school or clinical setting. As we shall shortly see, this has implications for how we understand what is occurring at the present moment.

Even within the university, the situation is somewhat predictable. Departments of philosophy are likely to teach bioethics as if there were no critique of the presuppositions of the mainstream position. The situation is more varied in religion departments, but even there it is possible to have mainstream bioethics taught as if it were the only alternative.

What, if anything, might we conclude? Surely religious voices have been marginalized, but just as surely there have been critiques about this within the academy. It may be that two or even more traditions of discourse will grow in bioethics; it is too soon to know what will happen. Tentatively, one might remain optimistic about the academic situation, in that alternatives are being argued for and about marginalization within academe.

11. Cf. Allen Verhey, "Integrity, Humility, and Heroism: May Patients Refuse Medical Treatment?" *The Reformed Journal* 32 (March 1982): 18-21.

12. Cf. Lisa Sowle Cahill, "Theology and Bioethics: Should Religious Traditions Have a Public Voice?" *The Journal of Medicine and Philosophy* (1992): 263-72. The theme of this particular issue is "Theology and Bioethics."

13. Cf. Daniel Callahan and Courtney S. Campbell, eds., "Theology, Religious Traditions, and Bioethics," a Special Supplement in *The Hastings Center Report* 20, no. 4 (July–August 1990).

The Profession of Medicine
and the Setting of the Clinic

Some preliminary remarks are in order. The evidence on the matter of marginalization of religious voices in the clinical setting is confusing. Indeed, I must say that one half of me, or better, that part of me that lives and works with physicians and nurses, was initially puzzled by the assignment to speak about the marginalization of religious voices in bioethics. The men and women with whom I work do not think it irrelevant that their patients have religious commitments, and they regard it as part of their task as healers to make sure these commitments are honored. Indeed, they often go to some trouble to do so. Nor do these men and women find it odd that persons actually want to live out their religious commitments, indeed, hope to flourish in doing so. One might claim, of course, that the religious commitments of the patients are the patients', and not the health care team's, and one might observe that respecting and taking care of patients who have religious commitments is different from admitting the patients' religious discourse into the physicians' and nurses' own conversations, especially when those conversations might make a difference about how they are going to act. However, within a clinical setting the patients' actions and words sometimes impress themselves on physicians and nurses, and can, in the quiet moments of medicine and nursing, be remembered and made a part of that world. But this is not all. The physicians' and nurses' religious commitments often become an explicit, if sometimes uncomfortable, part of the discussion. This is especially true in recent discussions of physician-assisted suicide and euthanasia, as well as in discussions of caring for HIV-seropositive patients. Thus I come to any discussion of this issue predisposed to be very careful in setting out judgments.

My first observation is simply that the marginalization of religious voices in bioethics in the context of health care is, well, odd. It is not just odd because initially religious voices were not muted in modern bioethics, especially when it came to discussions about what to do about particular kinds of cases, such as withdrawing treatment from terminally ill patients. It is odd because in the clinical context, although not in the public policy one, the reality of finitude takes on an immediacy that can be hidden from us in other settings. Academicians and public policy persons can operate as if finitude were an illusion or a bother; nurses and physicians do not have that luxury. Moreover, often enough persons who take care of patients hear "Why is this happening to me?" from patients who are not only speaking of physiological processes, but are also seeking some reason for their decline, disability, and illness — a reason that will allow them to make sense of their world. Physiological explanations do not give answers to these questions.[14]

Reflecting about medicine allows us to see an irony in all of this. Many who write in academic bioethics accept, or perhaps better, presume, the marginalization of religious voices, and this has had some effect on the non-academics reading their work — namely, physicians and nurses. The majority of clinicians are unaware of some of the methodological questions that bedevil the academics writing in this field. Thus the standard view of bioethics is taken for granted instead of understood as being challenged and questioned. The consequence of this is that most physicians and nurses do not understand how contested is the bioethics that they learn. Insofar as religious communities cooperate in this, they are misleading the very professionals they might hope to influence. That is to say, if one reads what I shall call the "clinical ethics" literature and the "academic bioethics" literature, something that I have to do, it is as if one is operating in two different worlds. In the academic bioethics literature, the very grounds of bioethics are at least sometimes challenged and subject to critique. In the clinical ethics literature, especially the clinical ethics literature now regularly appearing in medical journals, there is no attempt to bring the clinician up to date on the actual critiques of the kind of ethics that the physician is being asked to learn. Even the reviews-of-the-literature articles do not do this. In this sense, the writers of clinical ethics literature are not candid about the critiques that have been raised against the perspective that they presume to be

14. Suffering is also a topic that might have received similar discussion in the clinical setting. Again, the academy often pretends that it is not a topic for discussion, except to discuss how to eliminate it. For a noteworthy attempt at a discussion of this topic, cf. the articles in *Second Opinion* 9 (1988).

true. It may well be that they cannot be, for that would mean thinking about starting over again.[15]

Thus the situation in medicine is mixed. If one knows the academic bioethics literature well, one knows the standard paradigm, but one knows in addition the critique of that paradigm. By contrast, if one does not follow that literature — and this would apply to many practitioners interested in bioethics — one knows only the standard paradigm of the field. That paradigm has a certain power for practitioners for a fairly uncomplicated reason. The dominant paradigm of bioethics presented itself to concerned physicians and nurses as a form of universal reason, just as science so presented itself to medicine about a century ago. Physicians and others in medicine were attracted to a bioethics so presented because it was set forth as a moral framework for all persons. In its (pretended) universality it was like the science that had already been of such help in modern medical practice.

The profession easily borrowed this paradigm because it fit what health professionals had learned elsewhere. The physician supplied the medical facts of the situation and the patient supplied the values. Most of the time, this description appeared to serve both well. The physician had a limited but important domain, and the patient had a domain as well. Only when the patient asks for something beyond the limit of the usual is there a discussion.

Now, as I pointed out above, this paradigm of universal reason has been subjected to some critique by thinkers such as Alasdair MacIntyre, who argue that it is a particular paradigm of reason, that is, particular to this time and place in our Western intellectual history, and that its claims to universality — in that it attempts to escape that particularity — are nothing but pretension. If MacIntyre is correct, then the particular form of bioethics that has been brought into medical practice is a misleading one for the medical practitioner. It gives the practitioner the illusion that she or he is

---

15. The debates on euthanasia are opening up that possibility for nurses and physicians. Talking about respect for persons is often not enough. It is also the case that the famous Intensive Bioethics Course at the Kennedy Center has begun to offer alternative approaches to bioethics as part of its regular offerings. This is one place where the clinic and the academy meet.

dealing with universals, but in fact it speaks only to a particular time and place about what it is good to do or not to do in and through medicine. It is the particulars of time and place to which I shall turn.

In what follows, I am not making the claim that the marginalization of religious voices led to the situations that I will describe; the only claim is that the marginalization of religious voices did not help, coming when it did.

The paradigm of modern bioethics described above entered American medicine at a time when medicine was undergoing great changes.[16] American medicine was adopting the language of the market and the medical consumer. Under this model, the medical consumer, like the consumer in the regular marketplace, should not be challenged about his or her conception of a good life.

Unfortunately, this language of the market began to coalesce with the language of autonomy. One example of where this occurs is discussions of medical futility. For many thinkers, it is taken as a given that the principle of respect for personal autonomy settles the issue of futility. I refer to the bioethicists who argue that it is the patient's or the patient's surrogate's right to define what is futile for this patient, and if this is done in an idiosyncratic way, so be it. No one has the right to tell another what counts as a good life.[17] The patient's choice is immune from all public scrutiny. Courtney Campbell makes a point here that is worth keeping in mind. The emphasis on personal autonomy linked to the idea of privacy, in the context of market metaphors and models, delegitimates in a dramatic way

16. Cf. David J. Rothman, *Strangers at the Bedside: A History of How Law and Bioethics Transformed Medical Decision-making* (New York: Basic Books, 1991).

17. A theological commentary on the recent debate on medical futility would be the subject for at least one paper. For my purposes, it is enough to observe that the stronger the commitment to patient autonomy, the more likely the claim that patients and their surrogates have the right to demand medical treatment that physicians think is futile. In a recent example, Robert Veatch, well-known proponent of patient autonomy, defended a parent who demanded that a hospital treat her anencephalic daughter for respiratory distress. The usual treatment for anencephaly is comfort care, since ventilator support will not reverse or alleviate the underlying condition. Cf. Linda Greenhouse, "Court Order to Treat Baby with Partial Brain Prompts Debate on Courts and Ethics," *New York Times,* 20 February 1994, p. 20.

moral claims for not acquiescing in the autonomous choices of others.[18]

The coalescence of an emphasis on autonomy and a market model of medicine, with its implications concerning futility, cries out for critique, a critique informed by a different vision of medicine and of persons in community. To begin, it seems to me that we have disempowered persons in health care more than they ought to be. But that is not all. Health care personnel can and should remind us of one indisputable fact that we would like to deny: that we are mortal. But that is not all. Our purposes and projects, including medicine and nursing, are limited and finite. Given that they are limited, to attempt to use them past the time they may be of help is to turn health care into a false god, a technological idol that we worship. Instead, we have to understand the limits of what medicine and nursing can do. But still this is not all.

In my reading of my own and other religious traditions, one may not demand the use of resources that will deprive others of what is necessary for their flourishing when what one demands is not necessary for one's own flourishing. A society that tells us that we are to act like self-interested consumers and that acting like a self-interested consumer means getting all that you can for yourself at the lowest possible cost creates the circumstances that lead us into the current futility debate. Instead of thinking about our duties to others, we think of ourselves, and no one is empowered to tell us otherwise. If we have the funds, then we can determine the limits of our medical care; if we do not have the funds, then it is too bad, but we have no say. It is one of the unfortunate side effects of medicine becoming a business that it has lost the moral power it once had in people's lives. There is no sense that nurses and physicians might have anything to teach us about the limits of what might be accomplished through their disciplines. These very limits open up new possibilities of care, but they do not remove the impossibility of our living forever or the moral confusion that results when we attempt to involve medicine and nursing in that endeavor.

18. Campbell's point is made in the context of physician-assisted suicide and euthanasia, but it applies to the debate about futility as well. Cf. Campbell, "Principlism and Religion."

31

Furthermore, numerous commentators have pointed out that medicine — and here I focus more on medicine than on nursing — has lost some of its service orientation. This has not only been noticed by observers of medicine, it has been the focus of the laments of many of the older physicians who speak with me. Typical are the remarks of a Jewish physician friend of mine who is disappointed with many of the younger members of his profession. For this physician, to be allowed to go to the clinics and to practice medicine on the poor was a privilege not granted to everyone when he joined the medical staff fifty years ago. Now it is perceived by his new medical staff colleagues as a hindrance, something that one does, minimally, as part of being a member of the medical staff. If possible, one avoids it. It certainly is not a privilege. Along with this change of attitude toward caring for the poor has been the change of medicine to a business, with economic rationality and all that goes with it. Although there have been some comments on these matters, the way in which economic rationality starts to pervade medical practice and the corrosive effects this has on the ethos of medicine have to be lived with over time to be appreciated.[19]

I realize that one could attempt to explain these phenomena without referring to the marginalization of religious voices in bioethics. I also hasten to add that I would not put all of what has been happening within the profession down to a loss of religious voices. What I would claim is that insofar as religious voices have been muted or marginalized, the profession has lost a resource for self-correction that once was available to it. In short, the marginalization of religious

19. Let me give just one example. One of the things that has interested me in the time I have been working with physicians is the relative silence with which the AMA and ABA statement "Fifty Hours" was greeted, and the same silence that has greeted the AMA statement on "Caring for the Poor." I hasten to point out that I am not talking about opposition to the statements; what I am speaking about is the fact that the statements have been ignored. What might have been an opportunity within the profession to attempt to display professional commitments to the poor and underprivileged in this society has became another opportunity lost. Cf. G. D. Lundberg and L. Bodine, "Fifty Hours for the Poor," *JAMA* 258 (1987): 3157; Council on Ethical and Judicial Affairs, "Caring for the Poor," *JAMA* 269 (1992): 2533-37.

For a more extensive critique of the orientation of the profession toward economic paradigms and the problems it causes, cf. Marc A. Rodwin, *Medicine, Money, and Morals: Physicians' Conflicts of Interest* (New York: Oxford University Press, 1993).

voices has meant, in part, for the profession of medicine the loss of what James Gustafson has identified as the prophetic dimension of religious discourse, that dimension that challenges us to become what we might be but are not yet or asks us to remember what was and is not now.[20] I think Stanley Hauerwas is right when he suggests that medicine cannot correct itself on these matters and thus needs something like a church to remind it of what it might become.[21] The loss of the authority of this voice has, in my view, had unfortunate consequences for the profession.

This picture should not be painted only in one color. One only has to participate in discussions with nurses and physicians on why they care for patients who are HIV positive and a risk to their caregivers. This talk in hospital cafeterias displays all the ambivalence felt by physicians and nurses about their obligations to their patients. What remains is a fragment of what it means to be a professional, with obligations even in the face of potential danger to the self. That small remembrance might be encouraged and celebrated more than it is. But the marginalization of religious voices makes it difficult for these physicians and nurses to speak publicly about what keeps them going, even though they might admit it very privately in an aside. One of the difficulties for the profession of medicine is that, because legal and economic models have come to dominate, what remains of the sense of a profession, that is, of having something to profess, is becoming slim indeed.

Mainstream bioethics has been of little help in resisting this. We need to remember how bioethics came into the clinical setting — as part of a series of questions surrounding patient and physician prerogatives. It gave the patient a greater voice in making decisions, but it left aside other morally significant issues, including what should be decided and how resources should be allocated in medicine. Precisely at the point where medicine might have been held up to other paradigms, the only question became patient choice. It is no wonder that Steven Miles has criticized the ethicists in the clinic for their failure to call for a reform of medical practices. Indeed, at this point one can

20. James Gustafson, "Moral Discourse about Medicine: A Variety of Forms," *The Journal of Medicine and Philosophy* 15 (1990): 125-42.
21. Hauerwas, "Salvation and Health: Why Medicine Needs the Church."

use religious language in order to describe the activity of clinical bioethicists; they have acted as priests in the medical community, blessing the practices of the community without fundamentally challenging the presuppositions within which that community operated. Clinical ethicists resolve conflicts within the current practices of medicine instead of challenging those practices. The desire to be accepted within the medical community stands in the way of criticizing that community in an appropriate way.[22]

Students of religion would also be able to point out that different religions have also played this priestly role vis-à-vis institutions of power and prestige; this is not the first time in the history of civilization that this has been done. What is ironic is that it is being done by persons who wished often to exclude any religious voices from their world. Among other things, religious communities remember their own failure vis-à-vis centers of power. This, of course, does not mean that they always act on those memories.

One of the tragedies of the standard account of bioethics is that it is hard pressed to talk about the life of the professional. What brings women and men to medicine as a form of service to others, the enormous temptations to which they will be subjected because they can both do good and do well — this is attended to little or not at all. This might not be a problem if the limits of the standard account were explicitly laid out; unfortunately, up until now the discourse is too often presumed to be complete when these topics are not discussed.

There is a final, ironic consequence of the marginalization of religious voices in bioethics insofar as the profession is concerned. The law is left as the dominant source of morality for a profession dominated by persons who, and I choose these words carefully, often fear and sometimes despise lawyers. Ethics committees and institutional review boards, to use two examples, often worry about questions of legal liability before they worry about what it is right to do, or better, often their worries about what it is right to do are determined by their understanding of what their legal liability might be.

What might be concluded? First, religious voices are often marginalized in the clinical setting. Second, this marginalization has con-

22. Steven H. Miles, "Clinical Ethics and Reform of Access to Health Care," *Journal of Clinical Ethics* 4 (Fall 1993): 255-57.

tributed to the situation in which the profession is unable to speak about some features of professional life. Third, there is often no sense of the limited nature of the dominant discourse in bioethics and of what the alternatives might be. The fourth point is in the form of a suggestion. If there is to be a change in the clinic, this different discourse will have to find and/or develop a social location within the clinical setting. I have no wisdom about how that might happen.

Public Policy

The marginalization of religious voices has not taken place only in the academy or the profession. It is also occurring in public policy discussions. It is certainly the case, of course, that religious communities have been active in the public policy arena because of what they think are their own religious convictions. Thus groups that represent different churches have made many attempts to influence legislation. How they say what they say is another matter entirely, but one can hardly argue that religious institutions are not present.

Saying that religious communities enter into public policy discourse, however, does not tell the whole story, for the conditions under which they enter that discourse have an effect not only on how they say what they say but on how they are understood by the listeners. The focus of attention up to now has been the conditions for entrance, and there has been too little attention paid to how the churches will be heard, given the conditions of entrance. I will expand on these two issues.

There has been vigorous discussion on the conditions under which the churches and synagogues participate in public policy discussion. On what I have called the standard account, the language used cannot be the language of the particular religious community but must be the language of the larger secular community. In this case, what has been called the language of publicly accessible reasons means that the churches must speak the language or languages of liberalism.

Now a number of thinkers have focused on how this distorts the languages of the churches and synagogues. For example, the language of covenant does not easily translate into the language of contract. Thus there is a worry about how the languages of religious communities are inevitably distorted when they are forced to operate under the guise of the language of liberalism. One recent critique of this development is Stephen Carter's *The Culture of Disbelief.* Professor Carter, of Yale University Law School, argues that religious belief, qua religious, is downgraded and excluded from public discussions. Carter's argument is that religion is treated as if it were of no more significance than a person's hobby. Carter's complaint is quite strong: that religious belief is seen by some as incompatible with liberal democracy. Carter's concern is that religious institutions ought to be seen as independent centers of power and authority that are not subservient to the desires of the nation-state. The nation-state generally does not want to recognize alternative centers of power, and thus it tries either to trivialize religious belief by calling it private or to co-opt believers for the purposes of the state. Carter is not naive on this latter point. Too often believers are more than willing to be co-opted and to use the state's power for their own purposes.[23]

Theorists of the liberal state have argued that, although the state must be loathe to interfere with religious practices and has no jurisdiction over religious beliefs, the state may ask of all its citizens that if they enter the public sphere in an attempt to persuade, they frame their arguments so that all may understand and respond to them. One example of this kind of argument is found in Kent Greenwalt's *Religious Convictions and Political Choice.* Greenwalt argues that persons should use publicly accessible reasons for whatever claims that they put forward. This very much resembles the call for a neutral language of bioethics.[24]

Carter, however, is not persuaded by this call for a neutral language that all citizens should use. He agrees with Michael Perry, who argues that this demand handcuffs believers from being able to say what they mean in the language in which they wish to say it.[25]

Carter makes it clear that the marginalization of religious voices *in bioethics* is not the only marginalization of religious voices in the public

---

23. Stephen L. Carter, *The Culture of Disbelief* (New York: Basic Books, 1993).

24. Kent Greenwalt, *Religious Convictions and Political Choice* (New York: Oxford University Press, 1988).

25. Cf. Michael J. Perry, *Love and Power: The Role of Religion in American Politics* (New York: Oxford University Press, 1991).

policy arena. The marginalization of religious voices extends to any attempt to bring a religious voice into public discourse, and bioethical issues are just one example, to which he devotes one chapter. Although it may be a significant example, it is not the only one. Carter helps us understand that there is a wider context within which the marginalization of religious voices in bioethics occurs.[26]

Carter also reminds us that religious voices often enter into public policy discourse, even if they are often unwelcome. One of the interesting features of his analysis is the claim that religious communities not only do enter into the public discussion as communities, rather than as aggregates of individuals, but that they should so enter the public discussion. Carter's analysis presumes that religion is not simply the voice of an individual conscience, but an effort of a community of persons in most cases. One way to marginalize religious voices on this account is to insist that only individuals shorn of any connection to their communities can enter into the public forum. Carter would have us with our relationships in the middle of the conversation. Religious voices would not be privileged, but they would be welcome.

As helpful as Carter's analysis is, we should also note that the conditions of entrance into the conversation are not the only problem, and in many cases not the major problem, for churches and synagogues are not in the public arena in exactly the same way as other groups, or at least they might not be. Let me give an example.

When in the context of the debate about euthanasia in this country, some Jews worry about the cooperation of the medical profession with the Nazi regime in Germany during the Second World War, I take it that they are not in the first place worrying about Jews, but about the way in which a profession may be co-opted by what appear to be good ends and about the consequences of that co-optation. The reason they participate in the public policy discussion may not fit some understandings, under the paradigm of liberalism, of why groups participate in public policy discussion.

Under that paradigm people participate in public discussions in order to advance their own interests. When the churches and synagogues enter into such discussions, they risk being understood as operating in the same fashion as any other interest group. But even if

26. Carter, *The Culture of Disbelief,* 233-62.

the language that they use is the language of the public square, the reason they are there in the first place may well have to do with their religious commitments. To pretend otherwise is to misunderstand what might be occurring.

Now, of course, there is a problem. The problem is that the institutions are themselves brought under the banner of liberalism by assumptions about why they are there, namely, that they represent the interests of their particular religious communities. The interesting thing at this point is how the motivation of the actors is assumed to be known. Stripped, either by their own or by others' hands, of their ability to say in their own language what they might mean, they also lose the possibility for others to understand that they might be there for reasons that do not always fit the liberal paradigm about public discourse in liberal democracy. Ironically, it may be that the religious communities lose an important opportunity by not speaking more as to why they are present, as well as to the substance of the issue at hand, in their own language.[27]

The problems do not all lie in systematic distrust of the reasons for religious communities' presence and in the potential distortion of what they are saying. Religious communities are not always clear about why, from their own perspective, they are present. That is to say, to use the categories of H. Richard Niebuhr, are they there to stand over against culture, transform culture, or speak for the culture?[28] And even if the churches think they are clear about why they are present, it is not always clear to me that the way in which they choose to speak and act will accomplish what they wish to accomplish. For example, proponents of the church as an agent of transformation of culture should read Charles Scriven's account of the transformation of culture. Scriven's argument is that religious communities that aim only to witness might in fact have the most profound transformative effects, as opposed to those communities that imagine that by aiming at transformation they are likely to achieve it. It is not irrelevant to note

27. Careful readers will note that I am not arguing that religious communities always act in this fashion. On this point, cf. John A. Coleman, S.J., "Neither Liberal nor Socialist: The Originality of Catholic Social Teaching," in John A. Coleman, S.J., ed., *One Hundred Years of Catholic Social Thought* (Maryknoll, N.Y.: Orbis Books, 1991), 25-42.

28. H. Richard Niebuhr, *Christ and Culture* (New York: Harper & Row, 1951).

that these same communities of witness are less likely to be misunderstood because it is clear that they are not acting as an interest group when they speak to their own members about what kind of life the group should promote. Scriven, not surprisingly, focuses on the Anabaptists.[29]

The Roman Catholic tradition might well serve as an example of what Scriven might teach us. That tradition has had a long history of reflecting on the common good. That reflection presumed that the common good was greater than the sum of individual goods. When that reflection is carried over into the modern context, inevitably there will be misunderstandings. The assumptions of actors in the modern liberal state are that persons and institutions have interests and that only those count. The presupposition of the Catholic discussion (that there are goods in common that are prior to and greater than any individual good) is not shared, and inevitably people will be conversing at cross-purposes. More important for purposes of this discussion, transformation cannot take place under such circumstances. Another way of saying this is that the listener would first have to be transformed in order to be open to the possibility of discussing the common good, to begin to evaluate the claims being made by followers of the Roman Catholic tradition.

It is not being claimed here that churches never act as interest groups. What is at issue is whether there are times when it is possible to recognize that something else is at stake. If that possibility is systematically excluded, then inevitably there will be misunderstandings. In that sense, their voices are marginalized and will be even more so as long as churches and synagogues are not careful about their participation in public life in America.

We can summarize by saying that in the public policy arena there is a marginalization of religious voices, but there are also debates about how, if at all, religious people might enter into public policy discussions. Bioethics is one example of this in the public policy arena, and given the importance of many issues in bioethics, this marginalization is at best unfortunate.

---

29. Charles Scriven, *The Transformation of Culture: Christian Social Ethics after H. Richard Niebuhr* (Scottsdale, Penn.: Herald Press, 1988).

Conclusion

In this brief survey, I have not attended to many different activities of religious communities, activities that might provide further evidence that the marginalization of religious voices is not a single theme. For example, there is the work of the Lutheran Church of America, the Seventh Day Adventists — the list goes on. Nor have I highlighted the work of centers like the Institute of Religion and the Park Ridge Center in Chicago. These efforts focus primarily on what I have called the clinical or the public policy level, although contributions can occur at every level. Reading their materials can be enlightening, because one can often quickly identify the stresses and strains introduced into religious discourse by the predominant rhetoric of bioethics. Let me take just one example.

The Catholic Health Association was active in encouraging persons to fill out advance directives. During this effort, they used the rhetoric of personal choice. This rhetoric then had to be toned down when the Association opposed the Washington state initiative on physician-assisted suicide and euthanasia. Now, one can make reasonable and reasoned arguments for advance directives and against euthanasia. But in order to do this, one must spend some time speaking about freedom and dignity.[30]

On one level this paper may be understood as a lament, but on another I think it is a signal that it is important to attend to the criticisms of the standard bioethics that arise from within philosophy and from within the community of medical practitioners who are philosophically sophisticated. There is the beginning of a debate within academic bioethics that might be attended to by persons who wish to reinsert religious voices into bioethics. Specifically, these critics are suggesting that old questions, big questions as Maurice Natanson calls them, be addressed again.[31] And physicians are calling for dis-

---

30. The Catholic Health Association of the United States, *The Initiative 119 Campaign: Sharing Insights* (St. Louis: Catholic Health Association, 1992). In that document, it is made clear that it is important to avoid the language of choice in countering ballot initiatives to legalize physician-assisted suicide or euthanasia. Yet discussions of autonomy of patients depend on that language.

31. Maurice Natanson, "The Iliac Passion," *The Yale Journal of Biology and Medicine* 5 (1992): 165-72.

cussion of teaching and learning moral virtue. The particular locus of opportunity is the clinic.

I can imagine two different sorts of objection to this picture of marginalization that I have given. The first would argue that it is a particular piece of hubris for Christian thinkers or even for religious thinkers to imagine that their voices should be at the center of attention in bioethics. Although it is true that there were important voices influenced by religious traditions at the beginnings of this discipline, matters rapidly evolved so that philosophical categories, more acceptable to the majority of persons, become the dominant ones. If religious voices, especially Christian religious voices, wish to be at the center, they continue the illusion of Protestant America that Protestants should be in charge of things and ignore the fact that society has in fact changed. I hope that what I have said so far makes it clear that what I am lamenting is not the loss of Protestant hegemony in the discourse of this nation, nor am I claiming that religious voices should be at the center of the conversation. My discussion is about religious voices being a partner in the conversation.

The second sort of objection would celebrate the fact of marginalization. The claim here would be that it is a piece of foolishness for the churches to ask to be included in conversations in which their message will inevitably be distorted. Better to stand on the edges and witness to what they know to be true than to try to influence the larger society. When religious voices move to the center, they become co-opted by others who have no interest in religion and who use religion for their own purposes. Further, they become tempted to use force in order to impose their views, since that is what states, especially modern nation-states, do when they meet opposition. Thus my essay should be a celebration of the marginalization of religious voices in bioethics and not a lament for the current exclusion from the center of the public policy discussions. Marginalization gives the church freedom to do its business without worrying about how it will be received by the larger culture. From that vantage point, the church could critique a health care system and a profession gone seriously astray.

This last comment moves us into the discussion of what should be done. I must admit that this perspective appeals to me under certain circumstances, and it seems to me that it is especially powerful when one is dealing with the nation-state. I am not convinced that it is especially helpful when dealing with the profession and the academy.

What I am trying to reflect on here is my own Roman Catholic tradition and what I take to be an alternative offered to it, an alternative that suggests that we should turn our backs on the nation-state and bear witness without imagining that it is our task to influence the powers of this world. Both alternatives are possibilities if the circumstances are appropriate. It seems to me, however, that it is a mistake to argue that as a matter of principle the church should turn away from the nation-state, and that it is also a mistake to imagine that the church should remain an interested conversation partner with the state in all circumstances. Both positions of principle are mistaken. What is called for is some argument about the current situation within which religious communities find themselves and some assessment by those religious communities of their own histories on these matters. Thus, given different histories, different responses would be appropriate; what I am resisting here is a once-for-all solution to these questions.

All of this is going to become more, not less, difficult in the near future. My focus has been on the situation of medicine, for that is the situation that, in my view, holds the most promise.

For those who wish to enter the world of the clinic and the academy with a religious voice, dangers arise. The first danger is presuming that on a given issue a particular religious tradition has anything to say. Humility is in order. The second danger, related to the first, is not attending to other voices, religious or not. Listening is in order. The third danger is in assuming that discourse perhaps appropriate in one realm fits another. The medical community may be ready to hear discourse about virtue; I am not confident the academic community is as ready, even with all the discussion about virtue that we are reading and writing. That is to say, religious talk about virtue has as its purpose the creation of virtuous persons; it is not supposed to end in talk only. The irony is that on this particular subject, it may well be that religious communities will be asked to provide something that they cannot yet do, because they themselves have not been attending to the creation of virtuous people. Patience is in order.

But of course, these three activities of humility, listening, and patience would not be a bad place to begin, especially if one wishes to have influence in the clinic. These are among the activities necessary for a good nurse or physician, which is another way of saying that religious voices in bioethics should not worry only about voices, but about the activities out of which the voices speak.

Alien Dignity: The Legacy of Helmut Thielicke for Bioethics

KAREN LEBACQZ

This experience of rejection made me think that there was no God, because in moments of rejection like that one I feel I am no good. And if I am no good, how can there be any God? Am I not made in the image and likeness of God?[1]

With these haunting words, Ada Maria Isasi-Diaz points not only to the painful realities of racism and sexism in our midst but also to the centrality of the image of God for theological ethics and to the intimate link between that image and the valuation of human beings. "If I am no good, how can there be any God? Am I not made in the image and likeness of God?" What does it mean to be made in the image and likeness of God and how does it relate to our valuation as persons?

No modern ethicist has elaborated the link between the image of God and the valuing of persons with more care than the great German theologian Helmut Thielicke. Twenty-five years ago

---

1. Ada Maria Isasi-Diaz, "Las Palmas Reales de Ada," in Katie G. Cannon et al. (The Mudflower Collective), *God's Fierce Whimsy* (New York: Pilgrim Press, 1985), 106.

Thielicke provided the reflections on theological foundations for Houston's first international conference on ethics in medicine and technology. In "The Doctor as Judge of Who Shall Live and Who Shall Die,"[2] Thielicke suggested that there are two ways to view people: in terms of their utility, or in terms of their "infinite worth." Thielicke opted for their infinite worth, and based that option on his understanding of the "alien dignity" of persons.

In this essay, I will explore briefly the theological roots and meaning of "alien dignity" in Thielicke's thought, and then develop the legacy of this term for the task of health care ethics today by illustrating its implications in several arenas of medicine and health care. Although there are problems with the concept of alien dignity, I will argue that it provides a rich legacy for protecting and equalizing human beings, for requiring personal responsibility, for attending to structural problems in health care, and for seeing humans as fundamentally relational.

Alien Dignity and the Image of God

The "incommensurable, incalculable worth of human life,"[3] argued Thielicke, does not reside in any immanent quality of human beings, but in the fact that we are created and redeemed by God. Our worth is imparted by the love bestowed on us by God. Human worth is thus an "alien dignity," given in the relationship between humans and God. It is the image of God in us that gives us our alien dignity.

The image of God in humans was not, for Thielicke, a given attribute or property, such as rationality or even freedom.[4] Rather, "the divine likeness rests on the fact that God remembers [us]. . . ."[5] The image of God is not our own immanent or ontic dignity, not some quality such as rationality that "imitates" the character of the

2. Helmut Thielicke, "The Doctor as Judge of Who Shall Live and Who Shall Die," in Kenneth Vaux, ed., *Who Shall Live? Medicine, Technology, Ethics* (Philadelphia: Fortress Press, 1970).

3. Thielicke, "Doctor as Judge," 170.

4. Helmut Thielicke, *Theological Ethics, Volume 1: Foundations,* ed. William H. Lazareth (Philadelphia: Fortress Press, 1966), 151.

5. Thielicke, *Theological Ethics,* vol. 1, 165.

divine, but rather a statement of our relationship to God. To speak of the *imago Dei* is to speak of God's love for us. God creates us in love, calls us in love, and redeems us in love; and it is this love that creates the image of God in us and gives us our worth. The image of God is not substantive, but relational.

Human worth is therefore "alien" in the sense that it comes to us from God. It is "that alien dignity which is grounded in and by [the one] who does the giving."[6] As a *proprium,* a true ontic possession or attribute in the strict sense, it belongs only to Christ.[7] The divine likeness of human beings is fulfilled only in Christ. Only in Christ is there the immediacy of relation to God that constitutes the *imago Dei,* and that was destroyed in the "Fall." The immediacy thus lost is restored in Christ, and so we participate in this divine likeness through Christ. God "remembers" us and draws us back into proper relationship, and herein lies the image of God.

The image of God is therefore ineffable and difficult to describe concretely, since it does not consist in specific characteristics or attributes that can easily be named.[8] For Thielicke, the divine image in humans was like a mirror reflecting the glory of God. Like a mirror, the image goes dark when the source of light is withdrawn: "it possesses only borrowed light."[9]

The *imago Dei* is thus, substantively, a representation of agape — of God's love for humans. It is therefore also agape that recognizes and realizes the *imago Dei,* seeing the other person in her standing before God rather than in her "utility" value for me. It is agape that allows us to love our enemies, not identifying them with their opposition to us, but seeing in them the children of God.[10]

For Thielicke, then, to speak of the alien dignity of human beings is to speak of their infinite worth. It is to speak of their relationship to God, and of the love with which they are held by God. It is to speak of what God has "spent" on human beings, the love poured out that creates an unimpeachable worth possessed by "even the most pitiful

6. Thielicke, *Theological Ethics,* vol. 1, 170.
7. Thielicke, *Theological Ethics,* vol. 1, 171.
8. Thielicke, *Theological Ethics,* vol. 1, 159.
9. Thielicke, *Theological Ethics,* vol. 1, 177.
10. Thielicke, *The Ethics of Sex,* trans. John W. Doberstein (New York: Harper & Row, 1964), 32.

life."[11] To speak of alien dignity is to speak of the individual destiny received from God, of the indivisible totality of the person, of the person's standing in the eyes of God.

Problems with Alien Dignity

"Alien dignity" may not be a comfortable term today, especially for feminists and others from oppressed groups. Two problems are immediately evident. First, to speak of dignity as "alien" is to imply that it is not truly "ours." If the source is outside humans, then it seems something that is "not us." If it is only reflective of a light that originates elsewhere, then it seems that it could too easily be removed. To see dignity as "alien" thus seems to remove it too much from the *humanum* and to make it precarious.

In our post-Enlightenment world, and particularly since the human potential movement, the Western world has tended to stress the dignity and potential that are inherent to humans. We want a dignity that is *precisely* ours, that is so much a part of us that there can never be any recognition of us without an acknowledgment of that dignity. To suggest that one's dignity is "alien" and comes from outside may perhaps make us think that it is therefore more vulnerable to attack or erosion. We are probably more comfortable today with a notion of *intrinsic* dignity, as this notion would imply something so inbuilt that it can never be taken away.

Second, Thielicke's notion that alien dignity is like the reflection of a mirror in which all light comes from outside may appear to posit human beings as empty vessels. All value, all light, all dignity appear to come from God and from God alone. Thielicke's God seems distant and omnipotent. The gulf between the divine and the human seems virtually unbridgeable. Thielicke's alien dignity, the mirror reflecting God's light, seems to pose an all-powerful God and an all-empty human being: "the *imago Dei* depends on the reflecting of alien light, a process which is always under the control of the glory of God which casts the reflection."[12] Any sense of divine-human partnership seems

11. Thielicke, "Doctor as Judge," 172.
12. Thielicke, *Theological Ethics,* vol. 1, 180.

fragile at best. We appear to have a process in which humans are at most pawns in a game controlled by God.

Such a transcendent, omnipotent God has been abandoned in many contemporary theologies. Liberation and feminist theologians tend instead to speak of a vulnerable God who suffers with us or of a partnership between humans and God. How else are we to explain the suffering of children who are abused by their parents or of oppressed peoples everywhere? An omnipotent God who fails to intervene in human suffering seems a cruel hoax.[13]

We might wonder, then, whether Thielicke's notion of alien dignity is theologically and ethically adequate. Does it create too fragile a dignity, not sufficiently rooted in human nature itself? Does it pose a God too remote and removed for an age of liberation that needs a God who suffers with us?

Within the scope of this essay, I cannot fully address these questions. Nonetheless, I believe that such doubts may arise from a misreading of the implications of Thielicke's work, and that Thielicke's core notion of alien dignity offers protections and insights badly needed today. I will illustrate this claim by pointing to five implications of alien dignity and their application in bioethics.

Implications of Alien Dignity for Ethics

1. *Alien Dignity* Protects *People*.

That human dignity is "alien" does mean that it comes from outside me; it does not arise from within me. But for Thielicke, it is also integral to me. Since it is given to me in my very creation by God, since it is bestowed from the beginning with God's love, it is always present with me. It is therefore intimately mine, as truly mine as any of my characteristics and far more enduring. My youth will surely pass, my beauty will fade, but my alien dignity does *not* dim, in Thielicke's view.

---

13. See, e.g., Wendy Farley, *Tragic Vision and Divine Compassion: A Contemporary Theodicy* (Louisville, Ky.: Westminster/John Knox Press, 1990); Joanne Carlson Brown and Carole R. Bohn, eds., *Christianity, Patriarchy, and Abuse: A Feminist Critique* (New York: Pilgrim Press, 1989).

Precisely because human dignity is "alien," it does not have to be *earned,* and it cannot be *lost.* It does not depend on my skin color, my sex, my sexual orientation, my intelligence, or any other particular characteristic or achievement. It does not depend on "works."[14] Precisely because it is "alien" to me, it cannot be given away by me or taken away by others. It is both alien and inalienable. It is indelible, a mark put on us by God's love that permeates our being to the core. Since the alien dignity of humans depends only on God's love, and since God's love is constant and enduring, so is the dignity of each person.

To speak of alien dignity is therefore precisely a way of securing the basic inalienable worth of every person. Alien dignity *protects* people. They are inviolable. "Even the most pitiful life" retains its dignity, and its incommensurable, incalculable worth. Because of this worth, humans may not be subjected to the dictatorial rule of technical capacities.[15]

The concept of alien dignity thus provides a strong base for responding to difficult bioethical questions such as when to cease treatment. In "House Calls to Cardinal Jackson," David Schiedermayer struggles to explain why he continues to treat a 79-year-old woman who has been "mindless, lights-are-on-but-nobody's-home" for over ten years.[16] In trying to explain why he does not withdraw her feeding tube, Schiedermayer speaks of the daughter's love for the old woman and also of the fire that still burns in her green eyes. Then he asks:

> What is it that gives a person dignity? What is that inner grace that projects out toward the doctor, so that he, despite his intellect and education and training and skills, is taken aback? . . . The dignified are above reproach. You can't take dignity away from the dignified.[17]

Schiedermayer speaks here of the dignity of a woman who no longer functions as she once did. There is something about Cardinal Jackson

---

14. It also does not depend on faith, but only on the image of God. Thus, even the nonbeliever would have dignity.

15. Thielicke, "Doctor as Judge," 186.

16. David Schiedermayer, "The Case: House Calls to Cardinal Jackson," *Second Opinion* 17, no. 4 (April 1992): 35-40.

17. Schiedermayer, "The Case," 39.

that makes her inviolable to him, in spite of her advanced age and her mental incompetence. This something, which Schiedermayer calls her dignity, is what Thielicke would have called her alien dignity. For Thielicke, it is the worth that does not fade with age nor dim with incompetence because it comes from God.[18] Schiedermayer finds it harder to name the source of the dignity. He mentions not the love of God but the love of Cardinal Jackson's daughter, the hardship of Cardinal Jackson's life, the sense that we cannot abandon her after her history of discrimination and mistreatment.

While Schiedermayer does not name the same source of dignity that Thielicke would name, his understanding of the inviolability conferred by that dignity comes very close to Thielicke's. For Thielicke, alien dignity of humans means that others can never be treated simply for their instrumental value. They cannot be a means to an end for me. Their technical or utilitarian capacities do not define their worth. Hence, they do not lose their worth when they cease to function or when their capacities diminish.

In *The Ethics of Sex,*[19] for example, Thielicke argues against prostitution because it entails the instrumentalization of a human being. Such instrumentalization — turning the other into an instrument for my pleasure or satisfaction — is contrary to the alien dignity that prevents another from being simply a means to my ends.

Elsewhere, Thielicke argues that one can never fully possess another human being. To try to do so would be to destroy him at the center of his being.[20] One cannot split off parts of a person or objectify that person, but must deal with the whole person, with the "indivisible totality of a human being."[21] Only this is recognition of the alien dignity of the other.

Nor are others subject to the fickle nature of our emotions. To see another as the bearer of an alien dignity means that our regard for that other will remain even when her or his importance for us diminishes.[22]

---

18. Indeed, for Thielicke, her dignity would remain even if there was no fire in her eyes and no love proffered by her daughter.

19. Thielicke, *Ethics of Sex,* 33.

20. Thielicke, *Ethics of Sex,* 61.

21. Thielicke, *Ethics of Sex,* 63.

22. Thielicke, *Ethics of Sex,* 27.

Thus, in none of these ways can we take away the dignity of the other. Alien dignity protects the other from our vagaries, from objectification or instrumentalization, from our lust for possession or for power, from our imposition of our goals and purposes. If Cardinal Jackson's daughter tired of caring for her mother and ceased to love her, the old woman would not lose her dignity, in Thielicke's view.

In the medical arena, the inviolable worth of the other means that no one could simply be used, for example, as an organ bank. It means that research on human beings must respect those persons as whole beings, even if they are convicted criminals or the "most pitiful" of mental patients.[23] The notion of alien dignity provides fundamental protections against using persons as means to the ends of others, against objectifying people, against the intrusions of power to oppress the powerless.

2. *Alien Dignity* Equalizes *People.*

If the first implication of alien dignity is the protection of persons, the second is the equalization of persons. Since human worth is not earned or achieved, but given by God, no one is "worth" more than others. All were bought for a price, and therefore all carry an incalculable value. The worth of human life for Thielicke was "incommensurable" — it is not possible to measure one person's worth against another. Genuine agape, which recognizes the alien dignity in the other, "does not degrade the other person." Rather, it honors the other, and puts the other "on the same level" as the one doing the loving.[24] Alien dignity has an equalizing effect.

This is reinforced by understanding that alien dignity would never allow the other to be dealt with simply in utilitarian terms. The "use value" or "social contribution value" of the person is not the person's true value. Only the alien dignity, the love poured out by

23. See The National Commission for the Protection of Human Subjects, *Research Involving Those Institutionalized as Mentally Infirm,* DHEW #OS-78-0006, and *Research Involving Prisoners,* DHEW #OS-76-131.

24. Thielicke, *Theological Ethics, Volume 2: Politics,* ed. William H. Lazareth (Philadelphia: Fortress Press, 1969), 305.

God, represents the true value of the person. This value is unique, individual, incommensurable.

Operating out of this understanding of alien dignity would therefore prevent some approaches to the allocation of health care resources. In his study of medical directors of kidney dialysis and transplant facilities, John Kilner found that "more than half of the directors would assess the different social value of various candidates" for dialysis or transplant, and "less than a third would institute a more egalitarian random selection."[25] Thielicke's understanding of alien dignity would suggest that such attempts to measure the social worth of candidates for dialysis violates the incommensurable dignity of each.

In "The Doctor as Judge of Who Shall Live and Who Shall Die," Thielicke tackled directly the problem of insufficient resources to help those who might live with medical intervention. He recognized explicitly that at times, difficult choices must be made and some must be chosen to live while others die. Under these circumstances, humans will make the best choices they can. Considerations of social worth may in fact enter those choices. But there can never be, for Thielicke, an easy conscience about this choice. "One must simply run the risk of making the decision — and be prepared in so doing to err, and thereby to incur guilt."[26] When we must choose some to live at the price of death for others, we should experience that choice as wounding. These are the wounds that "must not be allowed to heal."[27] They touch on a deep "metaphysical" guilt that is built into the very structure of human existence[28] and that, ironically, makes us sound and healthy. Not to experience such guilt would be a sign that we forget the alien dignity and hence equality of all; to experience it is a sign that we recognize the alien dignity and equal worth of each. To do so is to be in partnership; thus, experiencing metaphysical guilt means that we remain fundamentally in relationship and hence healthy.

25. John F. Kilner, "Selecting Patients When Resources Are Limited: A Study of U.S. Medical Directors of Kidney Dialysis and Transplantation Facilities," *American Journal of Public Health* 78, no. 2 (1988): 146.

26. Thielicke, "Doctor as Judge," 166.

27. Thielicke, "Doctor as Judge," 173.

28. Thielicke, "Doctor as Judge," 164.

To say that alien dignity equalizes people is not to say that it makes everyone the same. The great diversity of human life is never denied by Thielicke. Indeed, he held to some traditional notions, for example of the differences between men and women and of the roles appropriate to them. But even in the midst of recognizing these differences, Thielicke held that women were right to demand respect because their alien dignity makes them "equal before God."[29] Women's different *roles* did not affect women's basic *worth* or *equality* with men, which is secured by their alien dignity. Similarly, people's different roles or status in life do not affect their basic value, which is secured by their alien dignity. Precisely because we are made in the image and likeness of God, we cannot be rejected as being "no good." Whatever our race, color, sex, class, or social status, we are all equal in the eyes of God.

From the notion of alien dignity, then, might come an appreciation not only of the protectability of humans, but of their equality within diversity. As the Human Genome Project continues to locate and define the many genes that make up human beings, it will be increasingly important to find a grounding for understanding equality in the midst of diversity. Our history of genetic discrimination indicates all too graphically how easy it is for human communities to establish genetic norms and discriminate against those who do not fit the norm.[30] As the Human Genome Project progresses, there is the danger that we will make judgments of social worth based on individual genomes. Troy Duster charges that we are opening a "backdoor" to eugenics, legitimizing social discrimination under the name of genetic science as we seek to correct "defective" genes.[31] Some will be judged not to have "normal" genes, others to have "superior" genes. Such judgments are exactly what the concept of "alien dignity" prevents. To accept diversity and yet affirm equality may be the most important challenge that lies before us in the realm of genetics. Thielicke's notion of alien dignity captures the underlying premise of equal worth amidst differing manifestations of human life.

29. Thielicke, *Ethics of Sex,* 12.

30. Troy Duster, *Backdoor to Eugenics* (New York: Routledge, 1990). See also John Horgan, "Eugenics Revisited," *Scientific American* 268, no. 6 (June 1993): 122-31.

31. Duster, *Backdoor to Eugenics,* 122-31.

3. *Alien Dignity Requires* Personal *Response.*

For Thielicke, the alien dignity of the other required an "I-Thou" relationship. Agape must be immediate, improvisational, non-routinized.[32] For Thielicke, there is no escaping personal responsibility by assuming that institutions or others will take over. The institutionalization of agape was therefore problematic: "Does not the Samaritan's ministry of mercy become inconceivable, is it not altered in its very substance, the moment it is institutionalized? . . ."[33] Thielicke cautioned against the "welfare state," because "no one is ever summoned personally" or need take personal responsibility in it.[34] In the welfare state, care would be "rationalized," and this very rationalization would kill the agape element in it.[35] Thus, the agape that responds to the alien dignity of the other, and in so responding realizes that dignity, must always be a personal response.

In the arena of health care, such a view may be an important corrective to the assumption that "others" or "the system" will provide. In the United States, for example, 95 percent of elderly people live not in nursing homes but in the community, dependent on care by family, friends, or hired workers. More than 80 percent are cared for by their families, and in 75 percent of these cases, the caregiver is a woman. Most of these women are over the age of fifty and not always in the best of health themselves.[36]

On the one hand, Thielicke would probably applaud these women. They have chosen positively, lovingly, and willingly to care for elderly spouses or parents. They exhibit agape. They assume personal responsibility.

On the other hand, the fact that 75 percent of the care is being done by women should make us ask, Where are the men? In Thielicke's view, no one should escape from personal response to and responsibility for the needs of others. A society that allows some to escape responsibility while others carry the burden would not meet

32. Thielicke, *Theological Ethics,* vol. 2, 291.
33. Thielicke, *Theological Ethics,* vol. 2, 291.
34. Thielicke, *Theological Ethics,* vol. 2, 292.
35. Thielicke, *Theological Ethics,* vol. 2, 294.
36. See Tish Sommers and Laurie Shields, *Women Take Care: The Consequences of Caregiving in Today's Society* (Gainsville, Fla.: Triad Publishing, 1987), 21.

with Thielicke's approval. Since Thielicke did not believe that a ministry of mercy could be institutionalized without losing something of its basic character, the institutionalization of caring as "women's work" or a "female function" might also violate his understanding of the need for personal responsibility. Thus, alien dignity could provide correctives to some societal arrangements.

4. *Alien Dignity Requires* **Structural Response.**

Thielicke's resistance to the institutionalization of care might be particularly problematic today for liberation theologians who stress the structural nature of injustice. It might seem at first glance that Thielicke's understanding of alien dignity would militate against nationalized health care or against a universal program such as that currently proposed by the Clinton administration. True, Clinton stressed personal responsibility in presenting his proposal to the nation. Responsibility is one of the principles presumably embedded in the design of the program.[37] Nonetheless, Clinton's program would require massive intervention on state and national levels to ensure access to health care for all American citizens and legal residents. Since Thielicke argued against routinization of care, one might wonder whether his I-Thou approach to alien dignity would undercut the Clinton plan.

Yet before we draw this conclusion, some nuancing is in order. It is true that Thielicke argued against the welfare state. The rationalizing or routinizing of care, he asserted, ran counter to what is characteristic of Christian love of the neighbor.[38] He was particularly troubled by the argument that the welfare recipient could "claim" welfare as a right, and that claiming such a right would be seen to honor the dignity of the person in ways that offering charity or agape does not.[39] But one must understand why Thielicke was troubled in order to understand the structural implications of his reflections on

37. *American Health Security Act of 1993,* Sept. 7, 1993, section 10 (Washington, D.C.: Bureau of National Affairs, 1993).
38. Thielicke, *Theological Ethics,* vol. 2, 300.
39. Thielicke, *Theological Ethics,* vol. 2, 304.

the welfare state. In spite of his reservations, his understanding of the implications of alien dignity pushes in the direction of a structural response to social and personal ills.

Thielicke's resistance to "rights" and preference for agape or charity was based on the understanding that love never degrades the other, but must treat the other as a true partner. "Rights" or claims separate people and force them into antagonistic relationships. Not antagonism, but a partnership "in the ultimate dimension" was, for Thielicke, the goal of all Christian action.[40] Precisely because of the alien dignity of the other, that other is meant to be seen as a person in the sight of God, never merely as an object. But if the other is a subject, contended Thielicke, then the other can never be left as the mere passive recipient of our actions. To do so is to degrade the other.

By the same token, poverty can never be accepted as the other person's fate.[41] The other must not simply be helped or sustained in poverty, but must "be restored to economic independence."[42] I have argued elsewhere that such restoration is implied by the Jubilee image of justice.[43] Such restoration requires structural undergirding. Rehabilitation was, for Thielicke, a proper undertaking of the state.[44]

In fact, for Thielicke the other must not simply be restored and helped to move out of poverty, but must be prevented from moving into poverty in the first place. "What is more urgently needed is preventive action."[45] Prevention, however, requires structural response: "a social order in which the right to gainful employment is assured and in which possibilities are created for the attainment of economic independence by way of education, financial credits, and the like."[46] Only such a structural, preventive response would constitute in Thielicke's view a genuine partnership or expression of agape.

Thus it is true that Thielicke argued for a limited role for the

40. Thielicke, *Theological Ethics,* vol. 2, 305.
41. Thielicke, *Theological Ethics,* vol. 2, 306.
42. Thielicke, *Theological Ethics,* vol. 2, 306.
43. See Karen Lebacqz, *Justice in an Unjust World* (Minneapolis: Augsburg Publishing House, 1987), ch. 7.
44. Thielicke, *Theological Ethics,* vol. 2, 307.
45. Thielicke, *Theological Ethics,* vol. 2, 306.
46. Thielicke, *Theological Ethics,* vol. 2, 306.

state and would not have condoned either the Marxist analysis or the more extensive welfare state supported in some liberation treatises today. At root, he understood agape to be a deeply personal response, and he shied away from any institutional response that would relieve personal responsibility. He feared the "impersonal machine" that would take away direct person-to-person care.[47] Nonetheless, his understanding of alien dignity also required preventive and structured response, in order to support the dignity of the other and the true partnership between people and between people and the state. Most significantly, it required not simply "charity" but moving people to a place of restored autonomy and self-support. Thielicke recognized the structural components of poverty and other human ills, and his understanding of alien dignity required attention to these components. To argue that the social order must guarantee a "right to gainful employment" is to take a large step toward structural justice.

By extension from this reasoning, I believe that we could also see in Thielicke's work the structural demands for a system of universal health care. If, as President Clinton said in his address to the nation, health care is crucial to the security necessary in order for people to make free choices and take risks for the future, then health care would be one of the structural demands of agape. Universal access to basic health care would recognize the alien dignity of all.

5. Alien Dignity Is Relational.

It is clear by now that Thielicke's concept of alien dignity is relational through and through. To have dignity is to be in relation.

First, it is to be in relation to God, who gives the dignity by investing love in people. Thus, one cannot speak of alien dignity without speaking of God's relationship to humankind. The very concept depends on relationality. Indeed, it connotes relationality, since for Thielicke alien dignity is not an "ontic" possession but precisely a statement of our relationship to God.

Second, to have alien dignity is to be in relation to people. It is others who realize our dignity by acting out of agape, out of a per-

47. Thielicke, *Theological Ethics*, vol. 2, 313.

spective of who we are before God. The term thus implies not only our "vertical" relation to God but also our "horizontal" relation to others.

Alien dignity is therefore very *personal,* but it is not *private* or atomistic. Dignity derives *between* beings — between humans and God, between humans and other humans. Thielicke called alien dignity "teleological, not ontological."[48] By this he meant that it does not refer to human characteristics or status, but to the purposes for which we are created by God. The term implies connections between beings and a fundamental covenant of life with life. To speak of alien dignity is therefore always to point us to relationship, interdependence, and covenant.

In this relationality, love is central. It is God's love that establishes the alien dignity of humans. It is human love that recognizes and realizes it. Once we know that God, like every mother, loves precisely the vulnerable and weak ones, then we know how irrevocable is the dignity of the poor and outcast. "If I am no good, how can there be any God? Am I not made in the image and likeness of God?" Our fate is not sealed by our actions or by the judgments of others about us, but by the love of God for us. Alien dignity is a Christological concept for Thielicke.

This notion of relationality also has important implications for contemporary bioethics. Criticisms of the current stress on "autonomy" are now legion.[49] Increasingly, bioethicists are searching for an approach to ethics that neither isolates the individual nor manufactures a false autonomy, but places the individual in social context, recognizing the role of family, of fiduciary relationships, of diminished autonomy. Feminists have been particularly keen on stressing caring and relationship as central to the tasks of ethics.

Thielicke's notion of alien dignity fits well with these concerns. Cardinal Jackson's dignity was not dependent on her mental capacity, but rather on her relationships. Significantly, as Schiedermayer struggled with what gave Jackson her dignity, he pointed both to past

---

48. Thielicke, *Theological Ethics,* vol. 1, 154.

49. See, e.g., Marshall B. Kapp, "Medical Empowerment of the Elderly," *Hastings Center Report* (July–August 1989): 5-7; George J. Agich, "Reassessing Autonomy in Long Term Care," *Hastings Center Report* (November-December 1990): 12-17.

relationships and to present ones, both to relationships of harm and to relationships of love. Cardinal Jackson's unassailable dignity came for him in part because of the love that her daughter still held for her. But it also came because a history of discrimination and mistreatment required a form of reparations — of refusing to abandon now one who had been abandoned in the past. In his own way, Schiedermayer attempts to establish a covenant that would assure Cardinal Jackson and her family that her dignity remained evident and appreciated. Cardinal Jackson does not have to have autonomy in order to be in relationship, to be the recipient of duties such as reparations on the part of others, to be loved and recognized. Her dignity — what Thielicke would call her alien dignity — is relational and implies covenant.

In response to Isasi-Diaz, Schiedermayer might say that the fact that she has experienced racist rejection in the past is precisely what gives her an inviolable dignity, just as it has contributed to that dignity for Cardinal Jackson. A relationship need not be one of love in order to remind us of the inviolable dignity of the other. Alien dignity requires a relational understanding of human life.

Conclusions

When Helmut Thielicke spoke to the first international conference on ethics in medicine and technology twenty-five years ago, health care ethics was in its infancy. The Human Genome Project, Kevorkian's "suicide machine" — these were unknowns. Abortion was not legal in the United States, in vitro fertilization clinics were not dotting the landscape as they now do. Much has changed in the intervening years.

Yet much has also remained the same. The genome project, assisted suicide, legalized abortion, in vitro fertilization — these modern developments raise ancient questions: should there be limits to human intervention in nature; when if at all is it permissible to take human life; should human bodies be bought and sold? At the root of these questions lies the ever present dilemma of the valuing of human life. What does it mean to be human, and what gives human life its worth?

It is to these foundational questions that Thielicke addressed his understanding of alien dignity. "If I am no good, how can there be any God? Am I not made in the image and likeness of God?" queries Isasi-Diaz. For Thielicke, being made in the image and likeness of God meant that each person gained an alien dignity that stamped a fundamental worth on that person — a worth so central and ineradicable that nothing done by oneself or by others could ever remove it. If there is a God, and if God is good, then so are we, for we are made in the image of God.

To be sure, Thielicke's precise formulation of alien dignity raises some problems. Although he speaks of partnership "in the ultimate dimension," it is not clear whether his understanding of alien dignity implies a true partnership between humans and God. His God seems distant and wholly "other," his human beings perhaps a bit too empty. Human dignity seems removed, perhaps a bit too alien.

Yet in spite of these problems, there is an enduring legacy here to which we would do well to attend. The notion of alien dignity provides considerable protection to human beings. It keeps us from being used as objects of others' desires or schemes and from being swept up in the instrumentalization of human life. This may be important for our consideration as we move toward increasing technological imperatives. Alien dignity also has a powerful equalizing vector, which may be important as we struggle to understand how to do ethics in the midst of diversity. Alien dignity requires both the immediacy of love and personal responsibility on the one hand, and on the other hand structures that undergird true partnership. It neither lets us off the hook nor reduces ethical action to mere sentimentality.[50] Finally, alien dignity requires a relational view of human beings. Such a focus on relationality is consonant with many feminist approaches to ethics, and provides an important corrective to the contemporary stress in bioethics on autonomy.

50. Some feminist texts that take "caring" or love as central to ethics do run the risk of dealing only with immediate relationships and failing to provide structural supports. See, for example, Nel Noddings, *Caring: A Feminist Approach to Ethics and Moral Education* (Berkeley: University of California Press, 1984).

How Christian Ethics Became Medical
Ethics: The Case of Paul Ramsey

STANLEY HAUERWAS

A Case

Beauchamp and Childress have just finished preparing the fourth
edition of their enormously successful *Principles of Biomedical Ethics*. It
occurred to me that someone ought to attend to the various redactions
of that book as we might learn much, not only about their own
changes of mind, but about the history of recent medical ethics. So I
asked Beauchamp and Childress if I might look at their files to see
what shaped and reshaped their revisions. Being old friends, they
graciously accepted my offer.

In the process I discovered a document that I think quite important given the purposes of this conference. It is a case that they
considered for inclusion in the famous appendix to their book, which
is simply called "Cases." Why they chose not to include the case, or
put pejoratively, why they may have suppressed the case, I expect to
be a matter of discussion for many years. I suspect they were thinking
about the case as a way to spark a consideration of the principle of
justice and they may have decided the case was too ambiguous, yet I
think their refusal to use the case involves deeper questions than
simply editorial relevance. Let me read you the case that bore the
number 666.

An elderly, but obviously quite active, man burst into a psychiatrist's office late one afternoon without an appointment. He seemed quite normal in appearance, though his ample sideburns made him appear a bit odd — like an academic left over from the nineteenth century. He said he had to talk with someone, because he suspected that his colleagues no longer listened to or could understand his arguments. He confessed he had little faith in psychiatry, but since psychiatrists were paid to listen he thought he might as well try one. This particular psychiatrist remembered that before the advent of psychotropics she actually used to talk to patients, so she decided to go along. After all, she had nothing better to do.

It was not immediately clear what was bothering the patient. Indeed, it did not seem to occur to the patient that he had become a patient. The psychiatrist in fact was a bit concerned whether the patient was stable, since there were some odd speech patterns accompanied by repetitive physical movements. For example, the patient kept saying, "You know," while pushing his finger into the psychiatrist's chest. There were also the constant "Hrumps" as the patient massaged his left chest with his right hand. He did all this while keeping his ever-present pipe going at full blast.

After some time the psychiatrist began to suspect that she had a case of serious paranoia on her hands. It seems the patient complained that no matter how hard he tried, few knew how to read rightly his many books. In effect he said he was suffering from the dread disease of chronic misinterpretation. For example, no matter how often he emphasized that he wrote as a Christian ethicist, people kept trying to turn him into one of the originators of the field of medical ethics.

He confessed that he had no brief against those who wanted to be medical ethicists, but his game was much larger — namely ensuring the moral survival of Christian civilization. After all, that civilization is the result of the Christian commitment embodied in such concepts as covenant fidelity, *hesed,* and agape. Such concepts often appear in the language of justice, duty, fairness, but in fact they are theological concepts through and through.

For example, some — in particular an undisciplined thinker at Duke — insisted on interpreting him in a Kantian manner simply because his book was called *The Patient as Person.* By *person* he certainly did not mean any Kantian account of "person," since that kind of individualism was exactly what he was trying to counter. After all, he did not title the book. The people at Yale did that. It must have been a liberal plot.

Moreover, most could not understand the relation, he claimed, between his views on war and the work he was doing in medical ethics. They thought his support of limited war inconsistent with his opposition to abortion. How could they fail to see that at the heart of each was his commitment to the inviolability of the individual? It is after all the neighbor, who comes in the form of individual human beings, that must be at the center of the Christian moral project.

The psychiatrist, after listening to these complaints, began to wonder what kind of diagnosis was appropriate. Was this really a case of chronic misinterpretation? The psychiatrist, of course, distrusted self-diagnosis, but there did seem to be a pattern emerging that might support such an account. Paranoia could not be excluded. In the absence of any strong evidence one way or the other, and feeling that the patient desperately needed calming, the psychiatrist, who had done a unit of CPE and discovered she had sadistic tendencies and that she ought to enjoy such desires, suggested that in the next week the patient read all of the *Church Dogmatics* and come back for a regular appointment.

Beauchamp and Childress ask provocatively at the end of the case, "Why is this case interesting?"

Christian Ethics and Medical Ethics

While I cannot pretend to explain why I think this case interesting, I do want to try to situate Ramsey's work in medical ethics, not only within his overall project, but in the history of Christian ethics in this country. Yet I have to tell you that my object is not to provide a better understanding of Ramsey, but rather to understand a bit better how Ramsey fits into the larger story of how and why Christian ethicists have become so fascinated with medical ethics.

I am currently working on a book that attempts to tell the story of Christian ethics as an academic discipline in America. The book asks the dramatic question, How did a tradition that began with a book called *Christianizing the Social Order*[1] end with a book called *Can Ethics Be Christian?* Gustafson describes his own sense of unease with the latter book, noting that he worked on the book for years "with the nagging sense that most persons who answer in an unambiguous affirmative would not be interested in my supporting argument, that a few fellow professional persons might be interested enough to look at it, and that for those who believe the answer is negative the question itself is not sufficiently important to bother about."[2] I suspect most of us concerned with Christian ethics and its relation to medical ethics are haunted by such an unease — who really cares?

Of course, Christian ethicists rushed into medical ethics for many reasons, not the least of which was and is money and power. I sometimes point out to my students that people now go to Europe to see the great cathedrals, wondering what kind of people would build such things — you might well be dead before the foundation was complete. Someday I think people may well come to see major medical centers like the one we have at Duke and ask what kind of people would build such things. If they are astute, they will think the builders certainly must have been afraid of death.

So medical ethicists, being the good priests they are, went to where the power is in liberal societies — medical schools. Kings and princes once surrounded themselves with priests for legitimation. Politicians today surround themselves with social scientists to give those they rule the impression that they really know what is going on and can plan accordingly.[3] Physicians, in an increasingly secular

1. *Christianizing the Social Order* was Walter Rauschenbusch's second book. The first was *Christianity and the Social Crisis,* which was published in 1907. The title of the second book suggests the extraordinary presumption that the social order could actually be "Christianized."

2. James Gustafson, "Theology Confronts Technology and the Life Sciences," *Commonweal,* 16 June 1978, 392.

3. Alasdair MacIntyre's account of the role of the "experts" in *After Virtue,* 2nd ed. (Notre Dame: University of Notre Dame Press, 1984) rightly argues that "predictability" becomes the legitimating category for rule in modern social orders. The distinction between "fact" and "value" is not epistemologically required but rather is produced by the necessity to create a social science that can ensure outcomes. The only difficulty, as MacIntyre argues, is that *fortuna* cannot be eliminated from human affairs (pp. 93-108).

society, surround themselves with medical ethicists. God no longer exists, the sacred universe of values has replaced God, and allegedly ethicists think about values and decisions that involve values.

Such an analysis may sound cynical, but I do not mean for it to be so interpreted. I simply assume such a development was inevitable given the character of our world. Nor do I mean to denigrate the good work of medical ethicists, who often take a quite critical stance toward the practices of those they serve. Yet the very terms of their analysis — autonomy, nonmaleficence, justice, and so forth — are primarily legitimating categories for a medicine shaped by a liberal culture. For example, it is by no means clear to me that informed consent necessarily should play the part attributed to it in most literature in medical ethics.[4] Given the Christian assumption that we are called to be of service to one another, I see no reason why some might not be drafted to be of help to one another — for example, to share blood — without their consent. Indeed, as I will show, Ramsey made such a suggestion.

That money and power have attracted Christian thinkers to medicine, however, is not the story I want to tell. Rather I want to direct attention to what might be called the "internal" story of Christian ethics, to try to understand how a tradition that began by trying to Christianize the social order now works very hard to show that being Christian does not unduly bias how we do medical ethics. Christian ethicists at one time wanted to rule, but now we seek to show we can be of help to the doctor. How did this happen?

I take my cue in this regard from Gustafson's wonderful article, "Theology Confronts Technology and the Life Sciences," that appeared in *Commonweal* in 1978. He begins the article by noting

> that persons with theological training are writing a great deal about technology and the life sciences is clear to those who read *The Hastings Center Report, Theological Studies* and many other journals. Whether *theology* is thereby in interaction with these areas, however,

---

4. I do not mean to suggest that informed consent is unimportant, but I think the account of autonomy that is used to shape accounts of informed consent distorts its use in medicine. For my attempt to provide a quite different account of informed consent based on friendship, see my *Suffering Presence: Theological Reflections on Medicine, the Mentally Handicapped, and the Church* (Notre Dame: University of Notre Dame Press, 1986), 114-24.

is less clear. For some writers the theological authorization for the ethical principles and procedures they use is explicit; this is clearly the case for the most prolific and polemical of the Protestants, Paul Ramsey. For others, writing as "ethicists," the relation of their moral discourse to any specific theological principles, or even to a definable religious outlook is opaque. Indeed, in response to a query from a friend (who is a distinguished philosopher) about how the term "ethicist" has come about, I responded in a pejorative way, "An ethicist is a former theologian who does not have the professional credentials of a moral philosopher."[5]

Gustafson continues by observing that much of the writing in the field of medical ethics is now done by people who desire to be known as "religious ethicists," if only to show they are distinguishable from philosophers. Yet it is by no means clear to what the adjective "religious" refers. It surely does not refer to anything as specific as "Jewish," or even "Protestant" or "Catholic," for if it did, the writers would use the proper designation. Gustafson commends Ramsey for his 1974 declaration, "I always write as the ethicist I am, namely a Christian ethicist, and not as some hypothetical common denominator."

I, too, think Ramsey is commendable for his candor. I am not, however, convinced that his execution matched his candor. I always kidded him that all the theology in *The Patient as Person* was in the preface. He did not find that remark humorous. He refused to let the more theological parts of *Ethics at the Edges of Life* be edited out, explicitly to rebut the criticism that *The Patient as Person* was insufficiently theological.[6] Yet it is not a matter of quantity but, rather, the

5. Gustafson, "Theology Confronts Technology and the Life Sciences," 386.
6. In the preface to *Ethics at the Edges of Life* (New Haven: Yale University Press, 1978), Ramsey emphasizes:

I do not hesitate to write as a Christian ethicist. No more did I hesitate in my first major book on medical ethics to invoke ultimate appeal to scripture or theology and to warrants such as righteousness, faithfulness, canons of loyalty, the awesome sanctity of human life, humankind in the image of God, holy ground, *hesed* (steadfast covenant love), agape (or "charity"), as these standards are understood in the religions of our culture, Judaism and Christianity. (p. xiii)

He continues on the next page to argue:

I go too far in apology. Such a reader will not find most of the following kind of theology that Ramsey represented. I will try to show that in spite of Ramsey's conservative reputation, both in theology and in politics, he remained ironically, like Reinhold Niebuhr, a theologian in the great tradition of Protestant liberalism.[7] Moreover, as a representative of that tradition he had insufficient resources to show how Christian practice might make a difference for understanding or forming the practice of medicine.

Ramsey in many ways was the last great representative of the Protestant social gospel. He could not, of course, call for a Christianizing of the social order. Reinhold Niebuhr had forever blocked that alternative. But Ramsey, like the social gospelers themselves, did not have to call for a Christianizing since he assumed that he was part

---

analysis to be parochially limited to a religious outlook. This is true for two reasons. In the first place, the Judeo-Christian tradition decisively influenced the origin and shape of medical ethics down to our own times. Unless an author absurdly proposes an entirely new ethics, he is bound to see ethical principles derived from our past religious culture. In short, medical ethics nearly to date is a concrete case of Christian "casuistry" — that is, it consists of the outlooks of the predominant Western religions *brought down to cases* and used to determine their resolution. . . . Whether medical ethics needs religious foundation, and whether it will be misshapen without it, awaits demonstration — or, more likely, the test of time. I do not undertake to argue the point. The humanist no more than I should want our opposite positions tested at such fateful constants. I do say, however, that the notion that an individual human life is absolutely unique, inviolable, irreplaceable, noninterchangeable, not substitutable, and not meldable with other lives is a notion that exists in our civilization because it is Christian; and that idea is so fundamental in the edifice of Western law and morals that it cannot be removed without bringing the whole house down.

In the second place, whether our moral outlooks are inspired by a humanistic vision of life or by a religious perspective, there may be a convergence between these points of departure on the plane of special moral problems.

7. Protestant liberal theology comes in many shapes and sizes. By suggesting Ramsey remained a Protestant liberal I am primarily locating his conversation partners — that is, the Niebuhrs. Ramsey's theological views were in many ways quite "conservative," but the structure of his own work assumed the results of Protestant liberalism. He, of course, read and appreciated Barth, but apart from employing the Barthian distinction between the external and internal covenant in *Christian Ethics and the Sit-In* (New York: Association Press, 1961), Ramsey never struggled with the methodological implications of Barth's work.

of a society that was well Christianized. Rauschenbusch could speak of saved and unsaved institutions, identifying the former with political democracy and suggesting that the economic order still needed saving. Ramsey would no longer speak of institutions being saved, but he certainly assumed that Christianity had formed something called Western civilization that bore the marks of the gospel. I think, moreover, it was no accident that given that presumption, medicine became a crucial practice that allowed him to develop that perspective. The church may no longer have social power, but at least we still have medicine.

One way to think about these matters is to consider what one thinks the subject of ethics to be. The social gospelers wanted to encompass all of life — economics, politics, family. With Reinhold Niebuhr the Christian ethicist's attention was focused less on economics — that would now be left to economists — than on politics, and in particular international politics. Ramsey's attempt to discipline some of the utilitarian presumptions of Niebuhr's realism can be read in deep continuity with Niebuhr's fascination with the world of international politics. But the problem with the focus on politics, and in particular international politics, is that it is just too messy. Medical ethics, by contrast, offers an opportunity for the kind of problems that could be casuistically displayed, thereby giving the sense that we just may know what we are doing when we do "ethics." Moreover, medical ethics, or better the practice of medicine, exemplified for Ramsey the moral commitments at the heart of Western civilization that do or at least should animate our politics and economics.

Ramsey's Understanding of the "Place" of Christian Ethics

I am aware that these are large themes, but let me try to suggest how this reading of Ramsey makes sense by calling attention to how his medical ethics fit within his overall project. Ramsey's basic theological position was set out in *Basic Christian Ethics*. He seldom returned to such theological questions, since he assumed that what he said there was right and needed no rethinking. However, he did write a quite candid essay about basic methodological issues in an article in 1982 called "Tradition and Reflection in Christian Life."[8]

In this article he confesses the following "puzzlement":

> Puzzlement is too weak a word. Disorientation is a better word, since I thrash about not knowing what to say to the present situation in the churches. For some time now the demise of the "Constantinian era" has been *triumphantly* proclaimed. We no longer live in "Christendom"; this fact is said to be abundantly clear. But why any Christian would cite this fact with joy I do not know. Still, that is not the heart of my puzzlement. My quandary is in attempting to understand how those who triumphantly proclaim the end of the Christian age can then still have the audacity to address pronouncements and counsel to governments. That was appropriate with the Constantinian era, not beyond, if we are beyond. Those who still address counsel to governments must believe *either* that a remnant of the Christian age remains on which they count when testifying before Congress *or* that in so doing they do so as only one among many other voices in a society that for the foreseeable future is irredeemably secular.[9]

I confess I love this quote not only because it is so quintessentially Ramsey in terms of its style, but also because he is so candid about his Constantinianism. Moreover, there is a wonderful footnote to the last sentence in which he identifies himself as one who still believes that a remnant remains of the Christian age that makes it possible for him to give counsel to government. He says,

> It is in this sense that I continue to try to do "public ethics." In this endeavor I have recently been put on notice that I may be wrong by a distinguished philosopher (MacIntyre), who wrote: "But any

8. Paul Ramsey, "Tradition and Reflection in Christian Life," *Perkins Journal of Theology* 35, no. 2 (Winter–Spring 1982): 46-56.

9. Ramsey, "Tradition and Reflection," 46-47. Ramsey returned to these considerations in his *Speak Up for Just War or Pacifism* (University Park: Pennsylvania State University Press, 1988), where he even suggested that "The hour cometh, and now is, when the practices accepted within Methodist hospitals may require the removal of the name 'Methodist' from them — if we are, with our physicians and health-care professionals, resolved to *be* the church of Jesus Christ" (p. 145).

biblical position, whether Jewish or Christian, is going to be at odds, so it seems, with the dominant secular standpoints of our culture; alliances between the theologians and the secular thinker are going to be limited to specific points or easily fractured by disagreements elsewhere. The modern secular world may provide fewer allies than Ramsey believes." At the same time I continue to try to do "church ethics" in hope that the day may come when the dominant secular viewpoints on morality will be extended from the church of Jesus Christ.[10]

Ramsey became increasingly convinced, at least if we are to believe some of his remarks in *Speak Up for Just War and Pacifism*, that the church might be forced to assume a sectlike stance. Yet he thought such a position was a matter of necessity rather than anything that Christians should want. For example, in a letter to me responding to my suggestion that his casuistry presumes that the notion of the inviolability of each life exists in our civilization because it is Christian, Ramsey says,

There are, of course, stretches in what we may dignify by calling my "special ethics" where the Christian word to be heard is not resounding in every paragraph. Call this Christian "casuistry" if you will — but not for the reason you state. Your grounds for my endeavor to do public ethics is partially true, as an appeal to *past* Christian influences perhaps not yet altogether lost. Doubtless I may hope against hope that some among the "hearers" may strengthen their adherence to the best of past culture; or maybe search among their premises and find that they have no breastplate of righteousness with which to gird the irreplaceability and unmeldability of every human soul. But I, the author, have not left Christian premises behind when I go on to do special ethics. You may *disagree* with the way I go about doing special ethics theologically, there where you say that my "dramatic and significant assertions" are only "assertions" for which no adequate theological warrant is supplied. I think everyone of them is adequately warranted, and *directly* by the "giftedness" of life. I judge that simple warrant to be enough. You may want me at this point to pause and retell

10. Ramsey, "Tradition and Reflection," 47.

the whole Christian story. But then we disagree more in style than in substance, for I never left that behind. . . . My foundational work is not [the humanist's] nor [the humanist's] mine. But I do believe that while Christianity ought always to be willing to be a sect whenever necessary, there is always at work a culture-forming impulse as well. When, therefore, I say I am disinterested in finding out whether the King is clothed, naked or wears a simple jock strap, I mean to say that Christian special ethics would still come to the conclusions I do.[11]

Indeed, it was in medicine that Ramsey found institutionalized the kind of moral presuppositions and practices that should be characteristic of Western civilization. Though he feared that we were in danger of having "a medical profession without a moral philosophy in a society without one either,"[12] it is nonetheless medicine, at least Ramsey's reading of medicine, that carries the Christian commitment to care for the neighbor as ensouled body. Therefore, the commitment of the physician to care for the patient prescending all other moral and social considerations provided Ramsey with a practice he sorely needed to sustain Christian ethics as a discipline in service to the world.

This, of course, involved two questionable presuppositions: (1) that Christians do or should attribute to the neighbor the significance Ramsey claims to find in the gospel, and (2) that medicine is

11. This letter is reprinted in the appendix of Steve Long's dissertation, "Whittling Off the Rough Edges: Paul Ramsey's Use of Just War Norms as Theory" (Ph.D. dissertation, Duke University, 1990), 318-19. My account of Ramsey's position owes much to Long's work. A revised and expanded version of his dissertation has been published under the title *Tragedy, Tradition, Transformism: The Ethics of Paul Ramsey* (Boulder: Westview Press, 1993). See pp. 207-8 for the quotation. I am indebted to Long for his criticism of this essay.

12. Paul Ramsey, *The Patient as Person* (New Haven: Yale University Press, 1970), 194. In a later essay, "The Nature of Medical Ethics," he put the matter even more strongly: "In an age, however, when ancient landmarks have been removed, and we are trying to do the unthinkable, namely, build a civilization without an agreed civil tradition and upon the absence of a moral consensus, everyone needs to be an ethicist to the extent of his capacity for reflection and his desire to be and to know that he is a reasonable person." This essay appeared in *The Teaching of Medical Ethics*, ed. Robert Veatch, Willard Gaylin, and Councilman Morgan (Hastings-on-Hudson: Hastings Institute Publication, 1973), 15.

or should be shaped by Ramsey's understanding of covenant fidelity. I will explore both these questions, for by doing so I think we will discover some of the reasons that Christian ethics has become medical ethics. Moreover, by looking into these matters I hope to substantiate my claim that Ramsey remained embedded in the habits of mind of liberal Protestantism as well as political liberalism.

Ramsey's "Ethics"

It is well known that Rauschenbusch thought Jesus was but the continuation of prophetic insight, since the prophets stood for a justice that was independent of cultic practice and religious dogma. What is important is not the "religious beliefs" but the ethical upshot. Ramsey was obviously infinitely more theologically sophisticated than Rauschenbusch, as well as personally more theologically "orthodox," but his understanding of the significance of "covenant fidelity" is structurally quite similar to Raschenbusch's understanding of the relation of theology and ethics.

For example, Ramsey, in a manner not unlike Rauschenbusch, thought the source of Christian life to be Jesus' preaching of the kingdom of God. But this presented a problem for Ramsey, at least when he was working on *Basic Christian Ethics*. Under the influence of Schweitzer, Ramsey assumed that the role of the kingdom in Jesus' teaching could not be separated from Jesus' eschatological expectations. "This has to be said, and so let it be said forthrightly: few contemporary Christians accept the kind of kingdom-expectation Jesus considered of central importance, and rightly they do not."[13] But if the kingdom is inseparably linked to an eschatology we can no longer accept, how can we continue to argue for the role of the kingdom as a source of Christian love?

Ramsey addressed the question by rejecting the avenue taken by Rauschenbusch and the social gospel; Rauschenbusch had read escha-

---

13. Paul Ramsey, *Basic Christian Ethics* (Louisville: Westminster/John Knox Press, 1993), 35-36. *Basic Christian Ethics* was originally published in 1950. This new edition contains a foreword by myself and Steve Long. Pagination to *Basic Christian Ethics* will appear in the text.

tology as if it simply named the inevitability of progress. In vintage Ramseyian polemical prose he writes, "Of course, it may be contended that apocalypticism is a better myth than the idea of progress prevalent since the eighteenth century, and New Testament eschatology at least permits a man to recognize a catastrophe when he sees one rather than dying in his procrustean bed of development with his illusions on" (36). Yet that further complicates his problem, for in a 1946 essay titled "A Theology of Social Action" he had said that

> we are correct, most especially, in no longer thinking as Jesus thought about the immediate end of the "this present age" and the coming of the kingdom of God. One of the main foundations and incentives for social action among us is the need for social control and some sort of restraint of evil to take the place left vacant by our rejection of Jesus' "eschatological" expectation.[14]

How could Ramsey reject the eschatology and maintain Jesus' emphasis on the kingdom's presence? He resolves this dilemma by claiming that the essence of Jesus' teaching about the kingdom, "disinterested love for the neighbor," was independent of its origin in Jesus' apocalypticism and stood on its own. In a passage that sounds as if it came from Bultmann's *Jesus Christ and Mythology*, Ramsey says,

> The origin and history of Christian love may be interesting and important in its own right, but to suppose that factors determining the origins of this conception have anything to do with its value, or affect its truth to any degree one way or another, is an instance of the "genetic fallacy" so prevalent in post-evolutionary thought.
> Indeed, precisely from the utter removal of all other considerations, Jesus' ethic gained an absolute validity transcending limitation to this or that place or time or civilization. Precisely because all other neighbors were apocalyptically removed from view except this single chance individual who might be hostile or friendly, beloved child or total stranger, Christian love gained unqualified lack of concern for either preferential interests or preferential duties, be-

14. Paul Ramsey, "A Theology of Social Action," *Social Action* 23, no. 2 (October 1946): 4. See further the foreword written by me and Steve Long for *Basic Christian Ethics*. This section of my account is taken from that foreword.

coming an attitude unconditionally required of men in spite of hostility, in spite also of friendliness, on the neighbor's part. (41-42) In short, Ramsey demythologizes apocalyptic and discovers disinterested love, which, though not exactly Kant, is at least in Kant's ballpark.

I need not tell you this was the center of his work for the rest of his life. We are always living in the end time when we face the needs of the neighbor. The unwillingness to subordinate the care of the neighbor to any other ends, even the ends of the survival of the human species, is the moral equivalent to living apocalyptically. Ramsey later recants his dismissal of Jesus' eschatology, but he never rethinks the structural presuppositions that come from his original account of neighbor love as absolute disinterestedness.

For example, in *Nine Modern Moralists,* in the midst of his discussion of Edmund Cahn and the ethics of the lifeboat, which in many ways was the basis for his later thinking on medical ethics, he seconds Cahn's judgment that the crisis in the lifeboat was apocalyptic in character. The lifeboat crisis, like Jesus' apocalyptic message, made null and void all earthly possessions, family ties, and distinctions of every conceivable kind. Accordingly, it embodies the ethics of the gospel that transcends the generic duty of self-preservation. Thus, love-transformed natural law requires that all should wait and die together rather than some lives be saved.[15]

Ramsey notes that this was the burden of Jesus' teaching, calling for an exodus from the natural order of existence to that made possible by the immediate presence of God.

> His ethics is not understandable apart from the presence of God's kingdom. It was not, as Schweitzer supposed, the imminent *coming* of the kingdom which produced Jesus' teachings as an "interim ethic." It was rather the *presence* of the kingdom which produced his unlimited estimate of what one man owes another in prompt and radical service; and at the same time it was his living in the presence of God which rendered negligible the fixed relationships

15. Paul Ramsey, *Nine Modern Moralists* (Englewood Cliffs, N.J.: Prentice-Hall, 1962), 248-49. In many ways *Nine Modern Moralists* is Ramsey's best book. See, for example, Scott Davis, "'Et Quod Vis Fac': Paul Ramsey and Augustinian Ethics," *Journal of Religious Ethics* 19, no. 2 (Fall 1991): 31-69, for a wonderful account of the significance of this book.

among men in this present age. His message does not stand or fall with his conception about the quick end of the world. It would be better to reverse this proposition and say that this expectation about the future sprang rather from Jesus' conviction about God and from Jesus' existence in his presence. Jesus and the prophets were so overwhelmed by their sense of the sovereign majesty and utter faithfulness of God . . . that the kingdoms, the legal systems and the customary or natural moralities of this world were already liquidated before their eyes. . . . Natural self-preservation was suspended, as also were the rules about Sabbath observance, if they stood in the way of manifesting the concrete response of serving the slightest need . . . of the neighbor.[16]

Ramsey adds a footnote to this passage in which he suggests that this paragraph significantly changes the emphasis, but not the "substance," of his interpretation "of the relation between eschatology and ethics in Jesus' teachings in *Basic Christian Ethics,* ch. 1."[17] I think that is certainly right; now Jesus' eschatology is interpreted as requiring us to act rightly though the heavens fall. Ramsey assumed that this was love-transformed justice that went beyond natural law and was not instantiated in the laws and practices of Western society. Indeed, I cannot help but think Ramsey's fascination with the law, which often resulted in painstaking (and pain-inducing) discussions of minutiae of the law, was the working out of his conviction that the gospel had transformed the *jus gentium,* making it necessary for the Christian ethicist to look to the law for the outworking of the Christian commitment to neighbor love.

Though Ramsey's account of neighbor love seemed to imply the protection of life as a necessary condition for our civilization, he never underwrote a survivalist ethic. Indeed, in his discussion of abortion in *War and the Christian Conscience,* he argues that a fetus in conflict-of-life cases should rightly be thought capable of sacrifice. For

the fetus is not only a man, with a right to life, but something of a Christian man who would not willingly exercise this right to the detriment of another, at least not when this abstract right is of no

16. Ramsey, *Nine Modern Moralists,* 248.
17. Ramsey, *Nine Modern Moralists,* 248.

advantage to him. Indeed, we should assume that *if* a fetus is capable of bearing rights he is also capable of exercising them in a charitable manner; and at the least this means that his own right to life should not be held on to in vain, to the detriment of that of another.[18]

It is an interesting question why Ramsey did not extend this line of reasoning to questions concerning experimentation on incompetents.

But why should this understanding of the "ethics" of the gospel be called Protestant liberalism? Quite simply, it allowed Ramsey to think that the nicer issues of theology — such as trinitarian and ecclesiological issues — were largely tangential to "ethics." Once neighbor love had been discovered, the ethicist could get on with the casuistry necessary for the working out of this commitment in Western civilization. As he puts it in *Basic Christian Ethics,* the problem is how Jesus' ethic of neighbor love can be transposed to a nonapocalyptic setting:

> What possible bearing can an ethic which specifies to the full what a man should do in relation to a single neighbor, an ethic which reveals with no qualification at all what the reign of "righteousness" means in regard to man, what bearing can this possibly have upon moral action in a world where *there is always more than one neighbor* and indeed a whole cluster of claims and responsibilities to be considered? (42)

I am not accusing Ramsey of the kind of reduction so characteristic of much of Protestant liberal theology — for example, Christ means love of the neighbor. Rather his position, in a sophisticated way to be sure, accepts the presumption that the gospel has a moral "upshot." The Christian "essence," moreover, has a kind of transhistorical validity because it is but an expression of the character of human existence.

Given this account of the "Christian thing," it should not be surprising that Ramsey would discover in medicine exactly the Christian commitment to the care of the neighbor. Nor is it surprising that the theology necessary for the work to be done in medical ethics could be stated in the preface to *The Patient as Person.* All that is required is

18. Paul Ramsey, *War and the Christian Conscience: How Shall Modern War Be Conducted Justly?* (Durham: Duke University Press, 1961), 182-83.

to assert that medicine but manifests one of the covenants into which we are born.[19] Medical care, in effect, is a love-transformed institution that is part of the Christian *jus gentium*. The major task for medical ethics is to reconcile the welfare of the individual with the welfare of humankind when both must be served.[20]

Ramsey, of course, thought this commitment under attack by atomistic individualism. Such an individualism erodes every bond of life with life — in particular the bonds into which we enter (spousal) and those into which we are born (filial). Moreover, the Cartesian dualism, that is, the strong distinction between body and soul so characteristic of modernity, creates the assumption that the quality of life can be separate from our bodily existence. Our individualism and Cartesianism combine to underwrite the Baconian project — "that is, the pervasive notion that, for every problem produced by technology used for the relief of the human condition, there will be an as-yet-distant technical solution."[21]

It is not, therefore, surprising that Ramsey shaped *The Patient as Person* around the problem of experimentation on children. Medical ethics is but the working out of the "ethics of consent." Experimentation raises the basic issues of fidelity between person and person.

> Consent expresses or establishes this relationship, and the requirement of consent sustains it. Fidelity is the bond between consenting man and consenting man in these procedures. The principle of an informed consent is the cardinal *canon of loyalty* joining men together in medical practice and investigation. In this requirement, faithfulness among men — the faithfulness that is normative for all the

19. In his fine article on Ramsey, "Paul Ramsey's Task: Some Methodological Clarifications and Questions," Paul Camenisch notes that Ramsey is not clear about the origin, authority, and content of the covenants under which we live. He suggests Ramsey vacillates between the view that the covenants originate at the will of the agents and the notion that the covenants operate outside the agent's will and are obligatory in themselves. I think Ramsey never thought this ambiguity needed resolution since he thought the crucial issue was the creation of a livable social order that respected the individual. Camenisch's article appears in *Love and Society: Essays in the Ethics of Paul Ramsey,* ed. James Johnson and David Smith (Missoula, Montana: Scholars Press, 1974), 67-90.

20. Ramsey, *Patient as Person,* xiv.

21. Ramsey, *Ethics at the Edges of Life,* 139.

covenants or moral bonds of life with life — gains specification for the primary relations peculiar to medical practice.[22]

It is not necessary to follow how Ramsey worked out this principle in matters of implied or proxy consent for the story I am trying to tell. What I hope is clear, however, is how Ramsey quite persuasively constructed medicine and medical ethics in terms of his understanding of the difference Christ has made. The irony is that it is unclear one needs Jesus' preaching of the kingdom for such an ethic. Yet, like a doctor who is more likely to find the diseases she has been trained to find, Ramsey made the primary moral issue in medical ethics the issue for which his ethics was designed. Moreover, in doing so he made medicine one of the fundamental carriers of his understanding of Christian civilization.

Ramsey's account of the ethos of medicine in *The Patient as Person* is so persuasive it is easy to miss what he fails to treat. For example, there is no discussion of the aims of medicine, what health or illness means or how they are determined, or the meaning and place of pain and suffering. Nor does he broach issues such as the economic and political presumptions that do or should sustain medicine. That he did not deal with such matters can be a carping criticism since no one can deal with every aspect of matters as complex as medicine. But the issue is not just that he did not deal with such matters, but that he could not, given his account of what "our ethics" should be.

I do not mean to suggest that such considerations are absent entirely from Ramsey's presentation of medical ethics. For example, his concern to free medicine from the secular understanding of death as unmitigated disaster is an indication that he sensed such issues mattered.[23] Yet how to distribute medical resources in a society determined by such a view of death is, according to Ramsey, virtually impossible. Indeed, he confesses he does not know how to answer questions of how to determine priorities within medical procedures or between medical procedures and other social priorities.[24] He calls

22. Ramsey, *Patient as Person*, 5.
23. Ramsey, *Patient as Person*, 269.
24. Ramsey, *Patient as Person*, 272.

for more mutual thought to be given to the setting of medical and social priorities, but observes,

> the expectation that this can be achieved is finally totalitarian, or else can only have a leveling or reductionist effect on the practice of medicine and on the whole human enterprise. We may perhaps know when priorities are decidedly out of joint; but no one knows exactly what are the joints. Civilization is simply not an arrangement of human activities in a set hierarchical order. A society is largely an unfocused meshing of human pursuits.[25]

This view of society is, of course, the view created by the great liberal theorists, who assumed that no teleological account of the universe and society was intelligible. Freedom is all that is left in such a world, but it is a freedom governed by no purpose. Consent is all we have to protect us from one another's arbitrary desires. The ethics of such social orders can be utilitarian or deontological, but both just reinforce and legitimate the more determinative social presuppositions. No doubt in some of his moods Ramsey resisted these presuppositions, but his account of neighbor love gave him insufficient resources to name or challenge this world.

I find it hard to see how it could be otherwise, given Ramsey's Constantinian commitments. Medicine, at least his account of medicine, confirmed his presumption that agape was in fact instantiated in Western culture. In effect, medicine became Ramsey's church as doctors in their commitment to patients remained more faithful to the ethic of Jesus than Christians who were constantly tempted to utopian dreams fueled by utilitarian presumptions.

Thus Ramsey's account of medicine is essentially conservative. He did not seek, as most liberals do not, to call into question the ends of medicine. Ends, other than the care of the patient, were simply not in the purview of ethics. Medicine, like the state, particularly the democratic state, was simply assumed to be the embodiment of love-transformed natural law. In like manner medicine was constituted by the deontological commitment he thought was at the heart of the gospel as well as our civilization. I am aware that Ramsey's position is more complex than the description "deontological" can compre-

25. Ramsey, *Patient as Person*, 275.

hend, but I find it hard to see how Ramsey takes us beyond what John Milbank has identified as deontological liberalism.[26] That such is the case should not be surprising, given the tradition of Christian ethics in which Ramsey stood. Christian ethics was destined to become medical ethics.

Medical Ethics after Ramsey

Where has all this gotten us? Not very far, I am afraid. I hope, however, it helps us understand why Ramsey, in spite of his strong declarations to be working as a Christian ethicist, prepared the way for the developments that Gustafson laments — that is, the subordination of theological ethics to medical ethics. If the social gospel prepared the way for Christian social ethicists to become social scientists with a difference, in many ways the more "orthodox" Ramsey prepared the way for Christian ethicists to become medical ethicists with a difference, the difference being the vague theological presumptions that do no serious intellectual work other than explaining, perhaps, the motivations of the "ethicist." As a result, Christian ethicists continue to leave the world as they found it. Why and how they might conceive of their task differently is a story for another day.

26. See, for example, John Milbank, " 'Between Purgation and Illumination': A Critique of the Theology of Right," in *Christ, Ethics, and Tragedy: Essays in Honour of Donald MacKinnon,* ed. Kenneth Surin (Cambridge: Cambridge University Press, 1989), 161-96.

Styles of Religious Reflection in Medical Ethics

JAMES M. GUSTAFSON

M ary Midgley wrote, "The main dispute in ethics these days lies between people who stress the *autonomy* of morals to avoid debasing them, and those who stress the *continuity of morals with other topics* in order to make them intelligible."[1] This is "the text" I elaborate on, respond to, and apply in this paper.

I have three points. First, there is a literature in Christian and other religious ethics, whether applied to medicine or other human activity, that assumes and defends the "autonomy" of religious ethics. This autonomy is justified on the basis of biblical authority, the authority of tradition, or the authority of religious institutions. Autonomous religious ethics then are applied to medicine.

Second, there is a literature in Christian and other religious ethics, whether applied to medicine or to other human activity, that interprets morals in continuity with other topics, for example, natural appetites and the human condition, in order to make ethics intelligible both within the religious community and beyond it. Religious ethics are described and explained, and their application to medicine is interpreted.

Third, there are those within religious communities who think that the explanation and interpretation of morals and the justification of ethics are interactive in a dialectical way.

1. Mary Midgley, *Heart and Mind* (Brighton, U.K.: Harvester Press, 1981), 131.

This is, in a sense, an ideal-typology. An ideal-typology is not a taxonomic device, into which various authors can be slotted, but a construct that, if it has value, has heuristic value. That is, it might help us to see tendencies in particular literature and, with more explication than I offer here, show how particular literature diverges from the ideal-type. A type, when properly used, ought to illumine the particularities of positions that in a general way fit it. Its use is to show the particularities of positions as illumined by the type. Much literature combines the three types I have isolated.

The Autonomy of Religious Ethics

First, the autonomy of religious ethics. Those who assume this mode are deeply concerned to maintain, in various ways, the integrity, identity, and particularity of a religious and theological position. This type can be defended in various ways, but it always makes a case for the distinctiveness, the specificity or singularity, or the uniqueness of the religious position — its authorization as a way of interpreting life in the world, its vision of the ends to be achieved, its standards of human conduct, and the depth of commitment it requires.

One defense can currently be backed by a general movement in intellectual and academic life, what used to be called the sociology of knowledge. All constructions of reality, as a whole or in particular aspects, are related to a point of departure that has a particular social, cultural, political, economic, or ideological basis. The playing field of disciplines, if not level, is more level than many attempts to achieve universal objectivity about what is known or believed. A line of critical inquiry, which historically had many of its origins in the history of modern theology, now pervades efforts to deal with everything from mathematics and physics to literature, religion, and morality. In its most radical forms, what used to be called presupposition hunting (something some theologians were quite skilled at doing with reference to other fields of inquiry) leads to the cacophony of intellectual and academic discourse, to not only relationalism but also extreme cognitive relativism. If this relativism is the case for the study of politics and nature, their claims for truth are no more secure than the claims made by a historic religious community — Christian, Jewish,

Islam, Buddhist, or what have you. Thus, in this cacophony of voices, it is legitimate for representatives of Christian and other perspectives and traditions to define their particularity and to join the noisy chorus in an effort to be heard. They have as much right as do rationalist moral philosophers, since the latter also are tradition related, if not tradition bound; all are partial and ideological.

Of course, debates continue about ethics not only among philosophers, but also within religious communities: which is the authentic representation of particularity to be affirmed? Within a more general justification of a religious ethics, and its right and responsibility to speak distinctively, arguments still occur as to which delineation of religious ethics is correct, or can best be defended. No one, to my knowledge, is willing to acquiesce to the judgment that all interpretations of ethics that can be denominated Christian or Jewish are equally plausible or valid. My point is simple: given the license to be particular, since everyone else is, some delineation of the distinctiveness is judged to be correct and others wrong, or at least one is better than others. Is the distinctiveness to be found in the rules of action, or action guides; or is it to be found in the interiority, the ultimate intentionality, of the agents? Is it to be found in the characteristics that shape the persistent patterns of outlooks and actions of the religious persons or communities, or is it to be found in the interpretations of the direction of the historical or even the cosmic process?

To use an overly simple rubric, "postmodernism" makes persons acutely aware of their particularities, and this can be accepted as an inevitability of thinking and acting. So, religious outlooks on medical and other activities are context related if not context determined. This being the case, rather than feel fear or shame for partiality, one can justify and affirm it. But among religious ethical writers, as well as others, some authorizations are sought to defend one interpretation of the particular to be correct, or at least better than alternatives. The arguments for criteria of evaluation within particular religious traditions invoke standards that back particular interpretations as the valid ones. A kind of autonomy for religious ethics can be justified on postmodern epistemological grounds, but within that autonomy some criteria of evaluation are used to defend more particular positions — between religious traditions and within each of them.

A second defense of the autonomy of religious ethics is a strong doctrine of particular revelation, whether to and through Moses, Jesus, or Mohammed. We have this defense stated boldly and flatly in evangelical fundamentalist ethics on issues of homosexuality and abortion, and more subtly and in mediated forms in other parts of Christianity (and other religious traditions). The general point is held by all traditionally orthodox theologies that belong to what have been called Abrahamic religions and ethics: God chose to be revealed to, in, and through particular persons or events that are narrated, reflected on, and authorized in some way by sacred texts.

This is the opposite extreme of the view I described above. Not historical accident, but truth is claimed for the basis of distinctive particularity, and thus the "autonomy" of theology and religious ethics. Because of this truth, the community and its ethical writers are bound to faithfully interpret the sacred texts.

Sometimes that leads to a specifically revealed morality, as in the Decalogue, and maybe in its application of the covenant and other biblical codes of morality and holiness. Christians make a distinction between the authority of the moral codes and the ritual or cultic codes. This implies either that there are some more general criteria that make the moral codes more authentic revelation than the cultic codes (see Aquinas, Calvin, Hooker, and many others), or that God intended the cultic to have a historical sunset clause but did not intend such for the moral. How such a revealed morality develops differs among religious traditions, and certainly within them.

One is impressed by the procedures of halakhic reasoning in the Orthodox Jewish tradition. A biblical text is examined for its biblical applications and their relations to other biblical contexts, and a tradition of interpretations develops that also is taken into account. Later codified forms and the interpretations of particular rabbis ascend to higher authority, so the work of a judge, or decisor, on a current medical matter is grounded in divine revelation and in knowledge of the interpretation of the tradition though a distinctive casuistical process. A life of holiness is fulfilled by conformity to the law; one is brought into the presence of God by obedience. Some Christians, quite to the contrary, isolate a biblical judgment and apply it directly to some currently proposed procedure. I think no more illustrations are needed with reference to revealed moral codes.

The choice of the distinctive center of revelation within sacred texts makes for differences in the revealed theological backing of medical and other ethics. For example, Barth's Christocentric theology leads both to different ethical procedures and to some different judgments from classic Thomistic or Lutheran ones. If the revelation centers on historical liberation one has a different basis for ethics from revelation centered on the cross, or on the mercy and forgiveness of God. The cosmic significance of Christ and the consequent *theosis* of Eastern Orthodoxy leads to different ethics from one based on the conviction that the life of the one in and through whom God is revealed also gives the shape and pattern of fidelity in human action. These differences, while all claiming fidelity to the revelation, can and do affect the norms and procedures of medical ethics.

In various forms of Christian, Jewish, and Islamic ethics revelation in the sacred text is developed through authorized strands of tradition, though arguments occur about the correct interpretation and elaboration. Tradition authorizes certain approaches to medical ethics, and to some particular moral precepts that are judged in some instances to be unexceptionable. The continuity of reflection through centuries creates a presumption of moral correctness; the weight of the argument is in favor of tradition. Dissent has to mount arguments from defensive positions. But tradition is not static. Development in tradition can be historically demonstrated in many cases, for example, as John Noonan has done in studies of usury, contraception, and other issues.

What backs the authority of tradition in religious medical ethics? One factor is the conviction that the distillation of ends and rules is the outcome of the thinking of those who are wise — always men until very recently. History seems to sift out what is judged to be wisdom from what is judged to be folly. Special authority accrues around persons and writings that have articulated procedures of thinking and moral ideas and ideals that are sustained by subsequent generations.

A second backing is communal practice, and not just ideas. Certain practices achieve the status of authenticity through time because they reflect fidelity to the revelation and apparently issue in activities and ends that are morally appropriate to the faith and beliefs.

Perhaps this is backed by a view that the Spirit, in Christianity, works through the thoughts and practices of both the leaders and the members of the community, guiding them faithfully through different courses of events and different circumstances. The autonomy of religious ethics is backed by the authority of tradition.

A third support for the autonomy of religious ethics can be institutional authority. Structures of power develop that authorize certain persons to speak for the revealed and traditional authorities. Means develop for the faithful to assess the degree of their compliance, and to have that compliance or noncompliance judged by empowered persons or communities. Authentic interpretation and application of revelation and tradition is sometimes controlled by persons in offices. If their power to allure consent and obedience is not sufficient, there are institutional means for enforcement and prescribed actions for bringing the wayward back into good standing. Or, in less formally authorized structures of power, more subtle forms function to gain consent and compliance. The autonomy of religious ethics is backed by the autonomy of religious institutions. The institutional guardians of the revelation and tradition, even when the tradition has been shaped by many nonbiblical sources, uphold and speak for the distinctiveness, specificity, singularity, or uniqueness, or at least for the integrity and autonomy, of a religious ethics.

I have not begun to show how these elaborations of Midgley's distinction carry over to medical ethics and how they are modified in their application. My basic ideal-construct is clear: religious ethics are autonomous, at least in the sense that they have an authorization that is specific to them. They are applied to medical matters; the traffic across the intersection to medical matters is basically in one direction. Alteration of the religious ethic by the findings of science, medicine, and other disciplines is resisted. This helps us to understand the medical ethical writings of many important Protestants and Catholics, and those of important writers in the Jewish and Islamic traditions as well. They affirm distinctiveness in some way, they claim some independence, and they are concerned to show how faithfulness to that authorization directs human conduct in medical matters. They are concerned not only to use that distinctiveness, but also to justify it.

The Intelligibility of Religious Ethics

Now to the second point. There is a literature in Christian and other religious ethics pertaining to medicine and other areas of activity that interprets morality in continuity with other topics to make religious ethics intelligible within and beyond the religious communities. Morality and ethics are explained; how they can be Christian or Jewish, or in some broad sense religious, is described. Thus religious ethics (or religious medical ethics) becomes intelligible; the intelligibility makes them understandable, tolerable, or even persuasive, especially if they add increments of depth or scope to what other views ignore or do not attend to sufficiently.

My addition to Midgley's statement is this: she takes the step of asserting that some scholars stress the continuity of morals with other topics. I take that step and another one, the second being the continuity between religious ethics and other ethics. Intelligibility is the desired outcome of both steps. Religious ethics belongs to the class of ethics; religion (Christianity, et al.) qualifies ethics to make it a subclass. I offer a few illustrations of this point.

First, there is a literature on how rules govern, or at least direct, decision making in many spheres of human activity and experience: economic, familial, political, legal, and so on. Thus there are all sorts of rules; to be governed or directed by rules is common in human experience. Morality shares with other areas of experience and activity the phenomenon of rules. But different from other arenas of rule-governed activity, or at least distinctive in its dimensions, is moral life. Rules can be distinguished that are moral in character, rather than legal or bureaucratic, or rules that govern social roles. Some position has to be taken on what distinguishes moral rules from other rules, and on that point there is not consensus. The discussion of that point is a subissue to what I wish to develop, and thus I will not expound it here. But morality is continuous with other "topics" in that it deals with a system of rules that govern behavior; to make this point makes morality intelligible in a certain context.

Religious morality, according to some views, is also a morality of rules. There is historical evidence for this: historic religious traditions have developed moral rules and moral codes. Some of these become legal in form because sanctions can be used against violators or because the procedures involved in their application are similar to procedures involved in different legal traditions. A rule, or a command, such as the command to love one's neighbor as oneself, is an example. Others are more specific in the actions they prescribe or proscribe. Thus, religious morality, or religious ethics, is continuous with ethics interpreted as rules.

What makes a rule of religious morality a religious rule? Again, there is no consensus on this point. It may be its presumed source: a command of a Deity; its presence in an authorized sacred text; its conformity to sayings and actions of a paradigmatic religious person; its source in a larger theological framework from which it is a necessary, or at least reasonable, inference with reference to the activity of those who accept the framework. The same rule might well be adhered to by nonreligious persons; what makes it religious is the particularity of its authorization or backing. It may be shared but have a particular obligatory force because it is part of a particular religious way of life. Or it may be a rule that is uniquely bound to its religious context, and adherence to it is seen as a matter of faithfulness to beliefs in that context; thus it might not be justifiable on any other grounds than its theological or religious ones.

A second illustration of the second point: Human activity is goal oriented; this is a descriptive premise, as is the assertion that human activity is rule governed. Negotiations between nation-states to reduce CFCs in the atmosphere have various proximate goals directed toward the reduction, if not elimination, of that pollutant. President Clinton's health care plan is goal oriented: he aspires to establish health care for all Americans. My faculty seminar is goal oriented; it seeks to develop understanding and intelligibility across academic disciplines. Morality is continuous with these other forms of activity and experience. It is oriented toward the actualization of certain ideals or ends. This view certainly has historic, as well as philosophical, backing.

Religious morality, according to some views, is also a morality of ends. There is historical evidence for this. The realization or approximation of ideal ends is an aspiration of many religious communities. One hopes for the day when the lion and the lamb shall lay down together; another is oriented by the symbol of the kingdom of God, which might be parsed out in terms of the realization of peace, justice, and the integrity of creation — to cite World Council of Churches language. Another is oriented toward some end of human wholeness, of which physical and mental health are ingredients. Thus religious morality or ethics is continuous with ethics interpreted as a vision or system of ends.

What makes an end in religious morality a religious end? Again, there is not consensus on this point. For some, the end of being human, individually and communally, is the vision of God; the realization of moral ends and values is an ingredient of the process that leads to that end. For some, since God is the creator of the order of life, there is a coincidence between realizing a moral determination of our natural ends and the fulfillment of human good physically and socially. For some the end is the lure and authority of a figure in sacred history; approximation in life of the significance of that figure is the end. The ends, like rules, might be widely shared, even though the reasons given by religious persons for their authority might be particular and distinctive. Or, again, there might be an end, for example, holiness in classic Judaism, that has a very particular religious authorization and might require particular forms of action to fulfill it. Religious morality of ends is made intelligible by its continuities with other ethics of ends and with other human activities. The intelligibility makes religious ethics at least understandable, and maybe persuasive, both within and outside the religious community.

My third illustration of the second point is the description, explanation, and interpretation of the "nature" of the human and of human activities. I mean "anthropology" in the classic sense: the morphology of humanity not only as distinct individual members but also as communities and a species. A decisive ingredient or dimension of every interpretation of economic, political, social, interpersonal experience, and of every commended or prescribed form of activity in these and other areas, is a descriptive anthropology. The description of the human in rational choice economics differs in some ways (though it may have similar outcomes) from that of sociobiology or psychoanalysis. In extrapolations from each of these endeavors to what is to be valued about life, there is coherence with its account of the human.

Morality is continuous with these endeavors; it shares some of their features. Thus we have different moral anthropologies: that of Aristotle is different from that of Kant; that of Hobbes is different from that of Rousseau; that of some feminist ethics is different from that of some male-dominated ethics; that of Enlightenment individualism in the West is different from that of Eastern traditions, which stress the interdependence of humans with all things and thus a priority of a common good. The moral anthropology is intrinsic to the determination within various perspectives of what range of considerations is morally relevant, what evils are to be avoided and what goods sought, what restraints are necessary on human activity, and what aims are worthy of commendation or approval. Ethics, like economics and other forms of activity and intellectual endeavor, is based on one or another descriptive and explanatory account of the human — individuals, societies, and even species. This helps to make ethics intelligible.

What makes a moral anthropology a religious moral anthropology? Again, there is not consensus on this point. One answer would be that its source of knowledge is the revelation in sacred texts and in traditions that are particular to a religious community. Thus, one can appeal to the Genesis statement that humans are made in the image of God. Or one can appeal to a Pauline text that stresses the universality of human sin. (I note that some economists have discovered "opportunism" and "the limits of rationality" to be sources of disturbance in economic institutions. This sounds like a rediscovery of sin and finitude to me.) Or one can appeal to a biblical text that makes claims for the restorative and redeeming power of the Spirit. The choice of a religious or theological backing for moral anthropology will affect how the moral life is interpreted: what is needed to restrain immorality, or to sustain and enhance morality; what the ends of human life are within which the moral is an ingredient or dimension. If Christianity, for example, is finally about redemption or salvation, how morality and ethics are authorized and delineated has to be correlated or be coherent with their relations to faith and theology.

Different religious traditions have different moral anthropologies, and these can deeply affect the interpretation of the human and its relation to nature, to society, and to the future. One recalls, for example, Arthur Danto's *Mysticism and Morality,* which seems to argue that within Eastern religions, and particularly Hinduism, the view of the human does not make ethics possible in a dominant Western sense.

Or, among many statements of a commonly made generalization, Joseph Kitagawa argues that "Eastern people have always accepted the humble role of being a part of the world of nature." "Gods proliferated, but they, like human beings and other beings, were subservient to the regulative order and inner balance of the cosmos, variously known as *Rta, Dharma,* and *Tao.*"[2] A larger and distinctive cosmological vision is the context for an anthropology; the moral anthropology is, at least in an ideal sense, saturated by this religious interpretation. The ethics that follow are framed and directed by the view of the human in the cosmos.

Moral or ethical visions or doctrines of the human are continuous with views of the human articulated for other purposes; religious moral visions of the human are made intelligible by showing their continuities with the concerns of any anthropology and by showing how the religion qualifies, adds distinctive dimensions, and the like, to moral anthropology.

Again, application to religious medical ethics is not specified in this paper. My general point is simple. Some literature in religious ethics makes such approaches intelligible both to members of religious communities and to others by explaining or interpreting religious morality and ethics in continuity with other ethics. This might make religious ethics persuasive, particularly if it has the power to disclose dimensions and features of medical care and morality that are opaque from other perspectives. The intersection with medicine or other areas is crossed, like my first point, in application, in one direction: from the side of religious ethics.

The Dialectic of Religious Ethics

Now to the third point, which goes beyond the quotation from Midgley, but follows the subsequent discussion of the polarity she draws. There are those within religious communities who think that the explanation and interpretation of morals and the justification of ethics are interactive in a dialectical way. This might revise religious and theological affirmations that are made, as well as the ethics and their

2. Joseph Kitagawa, *The History of Religions* (Atlanta: Scholars Press, 1987), 246.

91

applications. The authorization is not the autonomy of religious ethics, nor is the effort confined to making religious ethics intelligible. The dialectical interaction attempts to move from intelligibility to some kind of justification. And the recourse to religious language and symbols, and to theological language, hopefully broadens and deepens the interpretation of moral circumstances in medicine and elsewhere, and has some desirable outcome for the practices of morality in a human community more inclusive than those persons who can be socially identified as traditionally religious.

The interactional, dialectical process takes different forms, and it has different outcomes depending on the content of the materials related to each other. From the standpoint of my first point, for example, the articulation of a distinctively religious view might shed distinctive light on something about human life, in medical and other circumstances, that is persuasive because of its disclosive power, or because it presents a symbol that forcefully defines a critical conviction that is deemed necessary on other than religious grounds. An example of this would be the symbol of humans being in the image of God. The usual moral significance of this symbol is that each human being is worthy of intrinsic value and respect regardless of his or her particular conditions. The symbol is intelligible; while its authorization may be particularistic, its significance is presumed to be universal; it justifies a view of respect for persons. And in turn, though on somewhat different grounds, this view of respect gives an authority to the symbol. The symbol's rhetorical power is not just its source in sacred text, but its meaning. What is authorized by the "autonomy" of religious ethics is made intelligible; it is explained as to both its source and its implications. But it is also justifiable on other grounds, and lends a kind of authority to its usage in a wider community of discourse.

In the case of the idea of the image of God, the dialectical interaction does not necessitate any revision of the religious principle. But whether the image of God is reducible to the moral principle of respect for persons is questionable, depending on what other features of human beings theologians want to include in the image. And respect for persons can obviously be backed from Kantian or other views. But there is no fundamental clash between the two in some circumstances. In others there is, for example, in abortion debates and debates over death-delaying (usually called life-prolonging) therapies, where the judgments about qualities of personal or human existence differ.

The dialectic becomes critical in a culture that no longer adheres to a consensus about the theological or religious basis for respect for persons. In an essay, "The Sanctity of Life," Edward Shils states the continuing issues. The decline of Christian belief, he argues, is one of the major circumstances to be addressed in medical ethics. "The cognitive context of Christian doctrine, and above all the grandiose Christian symbolization of man's origin and destiny, have now lost much of their appeal."[3] Shils proposes a replacement. "The chief feature of the protoreligious, 'natural metaphysic' is the affirmation that life *is* sacred. It is believed to be sacred not because it is a manifestation of a transcendent creator from whom life comes: it is believed to be sacred because it is life. The idea of sacredness is generated by the primordial experience of being alive, of experiencing the elemental sensation of vitality and the elemental fear of its extinction" (p. 12). Thus he claims that life is sacred, "self-evidently" (pp. 18-19). The practical task "is not so much the re-establishment of Christianity . . . but rather the rediscovery of what it was that for so long gave such persuasive power to Christianity" (p. 38).

I restate this. The sanctity of life in our culture was explained during the dominance of Christianity by its coming from God. It is really grounded, Shils argues, in a universal and primordial experience of being alive. This "self-evidence" needs further justification, so he proposes a "natural metaphysic," which he does not develop. For Shils this is not merely an interesting intellectual and historical matter; it is critical to sustaining the value of the human in a secular culture that tends to erode it. The traditional ethic is explained historically in terms of a religion, then explained experientially, but what he calls a natural metaphysic, or what might be called a naturalistic theology of nature, is also needed. The traditional religious backing has to be revised; the dialectic calls for changing the historic religious justification, in order to be credible to many persons in our culture.

My point is that in the dialectical interaction between a religious

3. Edward Shils, "The Sanctity of Life," in *Life or Death,* ed. Daniel Labby (Seattle: University of Washington Press, 1968), 3.

explanation *and* justification of morality and ethics, and here particularly medical ethics, one way that some religious writers can and do justify ethics is by enlarging the scope of the "religious" so that persons no longer identified with historic religious communities can appreciate their own sense of the divine or sacred, and articulate it in nontraditional religious language, for example, Edward Shils. The dialectic calls for a revision of the religious traditions and a broader interpretation of aspects of their significance.

Some persons, like Mary Midgley, express this in a nonreductionist humanism. "Humanism," she writes, "exists to celebrate and increase the glory of human life, undistracted by reverence for any entities outside it. But as soon as we begin to cut away those entities, valuable elements in human life itself start to go, too. The center begins to bleed. The patterns essential to human life turn out to be ones that cannot be altogether contained within it. They must, if given their full scope, lead out far beyond it. To be fully human seems to involve being interested in other things as well as human ones, and sometimes more than human ones."[4] This begins a section entitled "The Chimera of Human Self-Sufficiency." Beginning with the human, and moving toward all the conditions necessary for its well-being, one makes a powerful case against human self-sufficiency. It does not, for Midgley, lead to theology, or to traditional religion, but it extends the boundaries to territory also interpretable by theologies of creation or nature. The limits of self-sufficiency — surely a point of theological orthodoxy — justify the expansion of the horizon and the territory to be accounted for. It is in that common territory that interaction calls for, to some religious thinkers, an articulation of bases for common morality.

The effect of such an interactional-dialectical interpretation of a basis for ethics clearly does not resolve moral quandaries in their specificity. But it does provide a backing — both in terms of a moral stance or attitude and in terms of some general principles — on which persons strongly identified with a religious tradition and others can converse about medical morality. It can resonate with the *sensus divini-*

4. Mary Midgley, "The Paradox of Humanism," in *James M. Gustafson's Theocentric Ethics,* ed. Harlan Beckley and Charles Swezey (Macon, Ga.: Mercer University Press, 1988), 193.

tatis that many persons not identified with the practice of particular religious communities have.

This paper is but a prologue to medical ethics. Authors, books, and articles could be named that have as central tendencies each of the three points, but to do so without intensive analysis and interpretation of these writings could lead to misunderstanding of my heuristic purpose.

It is important, in the end, to stress that each of these three ways of working has palpable limitations; something is gained and something is given up in each. My impression is that to some extent each of the points is taken with different colleagues and participants in mind. While there are serious intellectual issues to be met in arguing for the preferability of one over the other, in practice each is used, or all three may be used, depending on the occasions in which religious ethicists are engaged with others about what is right and good in various medical practices and policies.

A New Era for Bioethics: The Search for Meaning in Moral Experience

WARREN THOMAS REICH

with the assistance of Roberto dell'Oro

Several other chapters in this book look back to the beginnings of bioethics, and most approach bioethics from within a framework of theology or religious studies. My approach starts from within bioethics, and from within bioethics as a secular field of inquiry — secular in the sense that it is embedded in the concerns and dialogues of the world of our experience. All of the humanities and the life sciences contribute to this inquiry in an interdisciplinary way. I want, moreover, to turn attention from the past[1] to the present, to the crossroads that

1. I have documented in detail the birth of bioethics at conferences held in Padua (1990) and Seattle (1992) on the origins of bioethics. See Warren Thomas Reich, "La Bioetica negli Stati Uniti," in *Vent'anni di Bioetica: Idee, Protagonisti, Istituzioni*, ed. Corrado Viafora (Padova: Gregoriana, 1990), 143-75. (An English version of the book is forthcoming.) See also "The Word 'Bioethics': Its Birth and the Legacies of Those Who Shaped It," *Kennedy Institute of Ethics Journal* 4 (1994): 319-35; and "The

I acknowledge with gratitude the support of the Cleveland Clinic Foundation for research entailed in this work and for conferences at which the ideas were developed. I also want to thank the Institute of Religion in Houston and its former director, Allen Verhey, for providing me with a forum for testing and publishing these ideas.

bioethics faces now, and to the future, or at least to the direction in which, in my view, bioethics should be headed.

I want to argue for the importance of a sustained search for meaning in the context of ethics — a search for meaning that has been hindered in the medical context by the limited vision of positivist natural science, and in the framework of ethics by a preoccupation with the articulation and application of rules. I want to argue that this approach requires much more than simply "adding a little bit of meaning" to bioethical analysis and rule using. It entails a paradigm that functions, epistemologically, by turning first and primarily to experience and to the interpretation of experience — that is, to the discovery of the meaning of moral experience and the values and disvalues embedded in it — and then only secondarily to the study of the virtues, principles, rules, and practical judgments that embody this interpretation. I will examine several elements of an analysis of moral meaning, including the epistemological roles played by the ideas of care and attention, and I will illustrate the need for meaning in contemporary bioethics, suggesting an agenda for which the participation of theologians and religious scholars is crucially important.

The Divorce of Norm and Meaning in Bioethics

The problem of the search for meaning in bioethics is illustrated by the metaphor of the stethoscope. Richard Baron tells the story: "It happened the other morning on rounds, as it often does, that while I was carefully auscultating a patient's chest, he began to ask me a question. 'Quiet,' I said. 'I can't hear you while I'm listening.'"[2]

The "stethoscope metaphor" is emblematic of the inattention to meaning ("not hearing") in bioethics brought about by the reductionistic focus (the mode of restricted "listening") in the methodologies of both modern scientific medicine and contemporary ethical theory. The mind-set created by modern scientific medicine, whereby med-

---

Word 'Bioethics': The Struggle over Its Earliest Meanings," *Kennedy Institute of Ethics Journal* 5 (1995): 19-34.

2. Baron, "An Introduction to Medical Phenomenology: I Can't Hear You While I'm Listening," *Annals of Internal Medicine* 103 (1985): 606-11, at 606.

icine is strongly habituated to focus on ("listen to") diseases in an "objective" way, has required it to be inattentive to ("not hear") the sick person's experience of illness.[3] One can trace this mind-set historically to the influence of nineteenth-century medical scientists, particularly Wunderlich, Virchow, Helmholtz, and others, who proposed that practical clinical medicine be viewed as applied theoretical medicine. In this vision, clinical medicine came to be regarded as a source of questions to be addressed to a higher, theoretical discipline, pathologic physiology, which increasingly shaped clinical medicine. This led medicine to regard disease as an objective entity located anatomically or in a physiologic process. Careful scientific attention to the lesion or tumor has led to marvelous advances in modern medicine, but positivist natural science has also created a mind-set that has, in principle, excluded questions of meaning that are highly significant to human well-being and to the ethical aspects of medicine. Husserl pointedly analyzed the implications of this worldview:

> The exclusiveness with which the total world view of modern man, in the second half of the nineteenth century, let itself be determined by the positive sciences and be blinded by the "prosperity" they produced, meant an indifferent turning away from the questions which are decisive for a genuine humanity. . . . Fact-minded . . . science . . . excludes in principle precisely the questions which man, given over in our unhappy times to the most portentous upheavals, finds the most burning: questions of the meaning or meaninglessness of the whole of this human existence.[4]

What is needed is a medical mind-set that fosters the search for meaning — that is, the significance of illness, wellness, birth, dying, and so on for the sick or well person, for caregivers, for institutions, and for human society as a whole — in the context of an inquiry into moral values and disvalues, moral virtues and the like. A number of approaches have attempted to correct the medical mind-set and to move in this direction, including psychological, behavioral, and philo-

---

3. Baron, "An Introduction to Medical Phenomenology," 607-8.
4. Husserl, *The Crisis of European Sciences,* trans. David Carr (Evanston, Ill.: Northwestern University Press, 1970 [1954]), 5-6; cited by Baron in "An Introduction to Medical Phenomenology," 608.

sophical approaches. One such corrective approach is medical phenomenology, which shifts attention from the disease "out there" to the inner experience of illness "in here," where the real human experiences of suffering and dis-ease occur. This approach takes seriously perceptions of the world as experienced rather than accepting scientific descriptions of the world as exhaustive of human knowledge on the topic.[5] The goal is to reunite the "objective" and abstract world of science with the subjective world of human experience and its (objective) interpretation as meaningful or meaningless.

The "stethoscope metaphor" also symbolizes the mind-set of the moral philosophy that has dominated and shaped much of the first generation of bioethical inquiry. Bioethics has used its "stethoscope" — its instrument for auscultating the moral problems of the life sciences — to "listen" to a restricted language: the language of biomedical quandaries as well as that of the principles and rules ingredient in rational argumentation as applied to a determined case. The use of such a "stethoscope" strongly inclines one to be inattentive to significant moral voices that do not communicate in the language of quandary, do not create a challenge for ethical argument, or do not speak with the precision and articulateness that may be required in our intellectual culture for attracting the attention of serious ethical argumentation. Thus, both biomedical and ethical traditions have accentuated the problem of inattentiveness to the range of moral meaning that is significant and salient for moral reflection in bioethics.

The Methodological Shift Regarding Norm and Moral Meaning in Bioethics

A glance at the relatively brief history of epistemological developments in bioethics shows a methodological shift in the fundamental preoccupations of bioethicists. The scholars most commonly identified with being the first ones to elaborate a specifically bioethical body of literature — such as Paul Ramsey, Joseph Fletcher, and Van Rensselaer Potter — sought a horizon of meaning capable of sustaining ethical discourse that would respond to the value implications of technologi-

5. Baron, "An Introduction to Medical Phenomenlogy," 608.

cal developments in medicine and the life sciences. Those horizons of meaning — which inspired a moral-anthropological interpretive framework, whether theological or nonreligious humanistic — focused variously on the global moral meaning of nature, love, freedom, evolutionary progress, and so forth.

A major shift occurred at the end of the 1970s and the beginning of the 1980s. Under the increasing influence of contemporary Anglo-American moral philosophy, bioethics developed a preoccupation with the elaboration of normative criteria ("principles")[6] which drew their justification from the perspective of a restricted cluster of concepts in political philosophy. This moral philosophical approach sought to create a consensus based on shared arguments that were divorced from the horizon of meaning and the meaningful narratives that initially inspired them.[7]

This methodological transition can be understood as a step toward the development of a rationally consistent discipline. It constituted a sort of "secularization" of bioethics not unlike the trend of secularization and "demythologization" of theology that had occurred in previous decades of this century. It was religion that had constituted the horizon of ultimate reference, and provided the necessary conceptual ethical tools, for the interpretation of the delicate moral problems (such as human experimentation and allocation of health resources) that emerged in the first decade of the field of bioethics.[8] However, the religious foundations of bioethics were, to a considerable extent,

6. Confusion was caused by the use of the word *principles* (whose basic meaning is "sources") rather than *rules* to denote these moral criteria. For a comment on this terminology, see Warren Thomas Reich, "Introduction," in *Encyclopedia of Bioethics,* ed. Warren Thomas Reich, rev. ed. (New York: Simon & Schuster-Macmillan, 1995), xxviii-xxix.

7. I have analyzed the reliance of ethics and specifically bioethics on originary myths that create a horizon of meaning in "Alle origini dell'etica medica: Mito del contratto o mito di Cura?" in *Modelli di Medicina: Crisi e Attualità dell'Idea di Professione,* ed. Paolo Cattorini and Roberto Mordacci (Milan: Europa Scienze Umane Editrice, 1993), 35-59. Judith N. Shklar offered a thorough explanation of the reliance of ancient and modern political philosophy and ethics on creation myths in her "Subversive Genealogies," *Daedalus* 101 (1972): 129-54.

8. See LeRoy Walters, "Religion and the Renaissance of Medical Ethics in the United States: 1965-1975," in *Theology and Bioethics,* ed. Earl E. Shelp (Dordrecht, Netherlands: D. Reidel Publishing Company, 1985), 3-16.

couched in theoretical religious language, a major function of which was to elaborate a structure for religious (mostly Protestant and Catholic) identity, while also offering a moral vision intended to be useful for engaging in public moral discourse. Thus, by its very character, religious bioethics spoke in a language partly extraneous to the secular mind that was seeking normative guidance.[9]

Under the strong influence of the need for a consistent ethical basis for public policy formation, moral philosophy created for bioethics an arena of autonomous reflection by centering it on the use of principles (rules) and the ethical theory that unites them, especially deontological and utilitarian theories.[10] The clumsy term *principlism* is now used to designate this approach.

It is interesting that this philosophical framework has precipitated far more explicit and systematic criticism than the religious orientation ever elicited. I believe this anomaly can be explained only by viewing jointly the inadequacies of both approaches, for the inadequacy of the first approach presaged and merged with the inadequacy of the second. In significant ways, both approaches shared similar assumptions; in particular, they were both principally onto-theological in their approaches. Both were based on the assumption that the core truths could be expressed in a few basic concepts (or beliefs or principles), from which the remainder of ethics and ethical judgments would follow, by application and/or specification. Thus, while one (the theological) approach embraced a set of meanings, both approaches tended to exclude, by their a priori assumptions, the pursuit of meaning on the part of the moral agent.

Consequently, the parallel shortcomings of both approaches are illumined by the stethoscope metaphor. While "listening for" the place for the insertion of concepts of sin and redemption, nature and grace, moral principles and principle-like virtues, theology was disinclined to "hear" the voice of the molested and to "read" the complex implications

9. An exception is found in the writings of Richard A. McCormick, who utilized language that reached well beyond his Catholic community to address in a useful way a number of public policy issues in bioethics. See, for example, his *How Brave a New World? Dilemmas in Bioethics* (Washington, D.C.: Georgetown University Press, 1981).

10. Tom L. Beauchamp and James Childress, *Principles of Biomedical Ethics* (New York: Oxford University Press, 1979).

of new reproductive and transplant technologies. Freed of religious frameworks perceived as excessively sectarian in a pluralistic world, bioethics undoubtedly expected from the principles of moral philosophy an enduringly useful approach, only to discover — as noted above — that the stethoscope syndrome was found here, too. While "listening for" the signs and symptoms of the existence of quandaries to which its relatively few familiar concepts/principles could be applied, philosophy did not "hear" the voice and moral language of women, or the secular person's plaintive plea for the meaning of suffering, dying, and illness — a meaning that is crucial to moral decisions.

There are now, of course, a number of "alternative" approaches[11] to bioethics that, as I see it, have this in common: They narrow the gap between normative ethics and the search for moral meaning. But it is not my purpose to argue for an "alternative" ethical theory.[12] In fact, the conviction which is the point of departure for my reflections prescinds somewhat from the normative preoccupation that characterizes the development of an ethical theory. My conviction is that ethics finds its starting point and its ultimate formative element in an experiential paradigm characterized by the search for the meaning of moral experience.[13] Normative ethics — which proceeds, for example, through "application" of rules and the instantiation of virtues — occurs within this larger interpretive framework.[14]

11. The term "alternative approaches" is misleading, for it implies that the rule-based approach is fundamental and stable, while the other approaches — which actually account for the majority of the realms and levels of moral discourse — are reduced to being identified by that to which they are currently contrasted.

12. The various approaches that have not been sufficiently integrated into ethical and bioethical inquiry — and which I seek to unify around the central task of interpreting the meaning of moral experience — are nicely surveyed in *A Matter of Principles? Ferment in U.S. Bioethics,* ed. Edwin R. DuBose, Ron Hamel, and Laurence J. O'Connell (Valley Forge, Pa.: Trinity Press International, 1994).

13. I articulated this paradigm in "Bioethics in the 1980s: Challenges and Paradigms," in *Biomedical Ethics: A Community Forum,* ed. H. M. Sondheimer (Syracuse, N.Y.: SUNY Upstate Medical Center, 1985), 1-35. I developed the paradigm more extensively in "Ein neues Paradigma: Erfahrung als Quelle der Bioethik," in *Ethik in den Wissenschaften: Ariadnefaden im technischen Labyrinth?* ed. Klaus Steigleder and Dietmar Mieth (Tübingen: Attempto, 1991), 270-92.

14. European philosophical and theological language often uses the term *anthropology* (philosophical or moral anthropology) to incorporate the realm of meaning as "a necessary presupposition for the elaboration of normative criteria." See Roberto

It must be acknowledged that this claim about meaning raises a number of questions: Was there a "golden age" in which meaning and life were one — and if so, has that been lost in our culture? Was there a connection between the meaning of life and ethics in the classical worldview — and if so, what led to the loss of that connection? Is it desirable to (re)discover within contemporary ethical reflection the component of meaning? Isn't attention to meaning a luxury that in fact distracts from a pursuit of practical ethics? Even if it is desirable to retrieve the pursuit of meaning, why should we and how can we integrate the broader horizon of meaning into moral discourse, into practical moral judgments, and into our analysis of normative criteria?

A fleeting overview of responses to these questions, while not at all satisfying in their brevity, might at least help persuade the reader that meaning is, and always has been regarded as, an important part of human living; that reflection on meaning is an essential part of ethics; that ethics not based on the reflection on meaning is greatly impoverished and ultimately distorts the moral life; and that the ways of understanding moral meaning, as well as their certitude, change with various eras of human thought.

Recovering Meaning in Moral Discourse

In the West, it was the Greek mediation of meaning that resulted in classical culture — a culture that "breathed life and form into the civilization of Greece and Rome, . . . was born again in a European renaissance, [and] provided the chrysalis whence issued modern languages and literatures, modern mathematics and science, modern philosophy and history."[15] The Greek's world could be understood;

---

dell'Oro, "Antropologia ed etica: Oltre la bioetica nordamericana," *Rivista di Teologia Morale* 106 (1995): 203-20.

15. For these comments on the history and significance of meaning in classical and modern culture, I rely principally on Bernard Lonergan, "Dimensions of Meaning," in *Collection: Papers by Bernard Lonergan, S.J.,* ed. Frederick E. Crowe (New York: Herder & Herder, 1967), 252-67. Parenthetical references in the next few paragraphs are to this work. Lonergan also comments on the theme of meaning in his "Theology in Its New Context," in *Conversion: Perspectives on Personal and Social Transformation,* ed. Walter E. Conn (New York: Alba House, 1978), 3-21. See also Charles Taylor,

comprehension consisted in contemplating that reality and explaining it. For example, Socrates carried out an experiment that bears on meaning: In the early Platonic dialoges he put questions to the Athenians that had as their purpose moving them from the primary, spontaneous level of meaning — where humans employ everyday language, invoking, for example, notions like courage, justice, or self-control — to the secondary level of meaning, where they could say what they mean by everyday language: how to define courage, justice, or self-control (pp. 256-57).

Classicist thought interpreted and then standardized the meaning of the world in major concepts such as nature (*physis,* regarded as an original principle) and happiness (*eudaimonia* in the sense of the development of the essence of the individual). However, the same classicist tradition increasingly overlooked the lived and experienced dimension of human reality which is the constitutive function of meaning in human living.

A number of twentieth-century commentators have noted that, by and large, classical culture has passed away: "its norms of interpretation, its ways of thought, its manner in philosophy, its notion of science, its concept of law, its moral standards . . . are no longer accepted" (pp. 258-59). This breakdown is true of the meaning of both science and philosophy. By their very nature, classically oriented science and philosophy concentrated on the essential while ignoring the significance of the accidental, on the universal while neglecting the particular, on the necessary while belittling the contingent, on certitude while failing to see how tentative their theories were (pp. 259, 261).

By contrast, modern science aims to understand not just the essential but all phenomena; and it claims probability, not certitude, for its positive affirmations. Philosophy and other human sciences increasingly seek to understand not simply the essence of humanness (e.g., body and soul, matter and form) and the unchanging meaning of human nature with its correlatively enduring natural moral law, but what the classical worldview regarded as the accidental (such as family and other human relationships), the particular (the history of peoples,

---

"Theories of Meaning," in *Human Agency and Language: Philosophical Papers,* vol. 1 (Cambridge: Cambridge University Press, 1985), 248-92.

cultures, religion), and the contingent (e.g., trust as an indispensable yet contingent aspect of human moral growth).

Furthermore, classical culture conveyed the conviction that the literal meaning of words and phrases somehow has priority, while figurative meaning is an ornament that makes the literal meaning more vivid and effective. Giambattista Vico is renowned for having put forward, in his *Scienza nuova,* the contrary view by proclaiming the priority of poetry. To proclaim the priority of poetry — and/or the priority of imagination — is a way of confirming that humans come to know and to express themselves through symbol and imagination before they know and can express conceptually (if ever they come to know and express conceptually) what these symbols literally mean. Much of the contemporary turn to inquiry into the meaning of experience is dependent on this question of the priority and role of preconceptual, imaginative language. Heeding the role of meaning has long been made difficult by the widespread philosophical assumption that since the Enlightenment one must divorce reason from both imagination and emotion. Yet even some of the leading Enlightenment philosophers quickly acknowledged that imagination is inherent in all knowledge and reasoning; and contemporary thought increasingly acknowledges the essential role of emotion and sentiment in human knowledge in general and the quest for meaning in particular.

The meaning and function of ethics have undergone the same stages in their development and ultimately the same recent shift in paradigm as have science, philosophy, and the other disciplines. So-called classical moral reflection — inspired by Aristotelianism and subsequently by medieval Thomism — was, by definition, a reflection on meaning: It proposed that reflection on the immediate criteria for acting was secondary in respect to the identification of a *telos* to be pursued.[16] In Aristotelian ethics, fundamental attention was not given primarily to concrete action and the norms that regulate it, but given more globally to the *praxis* that covers an entire existence and defines the destiny of life.[17] The good is only secondarily a law to be applied in a concrete case;

16. The theoretically complex history of the resistance of ethics to the question of meaning is traced by Alasdair MacIntyre in *After Virtue: A Study in Moral Theory,* 2nd ed. (Notre Dame: University of Notre Dame Press, 1984).

17. See Hans-Georg Gadamer, *The Idea of the Good in the Platonic-Aristotelian Philosophy,* trans. P. Christopher Smith (New Haven: Yale University Press, 1986).

primum et per se, it is the very horizon of the choices with which the agent designs his or her own moral space and the ultimate measure of his or her actions. The good bears the weight of individual moral decisions and unifies their meaning in the coherence of an overriding vision. This coherence can be seen only dimly and pursued with the liberty of a project, not with the cogent evidence of a mathematical formula. Yet, over time, classical ethics developed a deep cleavage. To make the notion of good applicable in both philosophical and theological contexts, it developed principles and principle-like virtues whose formal philosophical function adopted more and more the characteristics of precision and certitude; yet their meaning was not precise, for ethics, regarded as practical science, is none other than the uncertain measure of freedom in the complexity of life.[18]

The classical era was an era in which meaning was commonly perceived and peacefully shared. Ethics was able to point the way to the realization of an end the truth of which was already established, for the *polis* or *societas christiana* did not yet know the split imposed by ideological pluralism. The modern epoch, which was born under the sign of religious division and anthropological pessimism, developed an ethic symbolized by a Hobbesian vision of all humans warring against all others. The purpose of ethics came to be the achievement of harmony and the promise of peace. Rational argumentation pertaining to a cluster of univocal ethical criteria that were to be universally applied came to represent the only significant purpose of moral reflection.[19] Indeed, following the Hobbesian vision of social chaos and the need for social consensus regarding coercive restraints, Engelhardt reduces the substantive content of ethics (and bioethics) to freedom/autonomy.[20]

18. Note Aristotle's explanation of ethics in the *Nichomachean Ethics,* trans. William David Ross (New York: Random House, 1941), and how it is viewed by Charles Taylor in his *Sources of the Self: The Making of Modern Identity* (Cambridge, Mass.: Harvard University Press, 1989).

19. See Hans-Georg Gadamer, *Über die Möglichkeit einer philosophischen Ethik,* in *Kleine Schriften* (Tübingen: 1967), vol. 1, 179-91. On the fundamentally different starting-points of "classical" and "modern" ethics, see also the instructive reflections of Ernst Tugendhat in *Probleme der Ethik* (Stuttgart: 1984).

20. H. Tristram Engelhardt Jr., *The Foundations of Bioethics* (New York: Oxford University Press, 1986).

In fact, however, modern ethics has been bracketed by meaning: Human experience has remained inscribed in the horizon of meaning and the individual conscience manifested the lived moral meaning of all individuals; but neither locus of moral meaning could find its way into philosophical ethics, for neither was judged amenable to public moral discourse. Increasingly distanced from the major frameworks for meaning that were found in the classical era's natural teleology for the good and its religious eudaemonism, modern ethics came to restrict itself minimally to the mere metaethical meaning of moral language itself,[21] and maximally to moral argumentation that was universally valid but significantly void of the content of moral meaning that might serve to articulate a web of socially shared convictions.[22]

The severely problematic question of the current direction to be taken by ethics and bioethics in particular arises from the situation in which ethics has increasingly become characterized by a rationality turned instrumental, due to the conviction that the pursuit of moral meaning is superfluous to the ethical enterprise. What is at stake in our choice of ethical roads to be taken in the next era of bioethics — and ethics more generally — is the very nature of moral reflection.

Retrieving the Pursuit of Meaning in the Practice of Contemporary Bioethics

The foregoing, brief historical survey highlights the importance of the recurring conviction that moral reflection does not begin with the analysis of arguments dealing with rules — that is, with normative

21. See, for example, Richard M. Hare, *Moral Thinking: Its Levels, Method, and Point* (Oxford: Clarendon Press, 1981).

22. I say "significantly" but not totally, because the ethical scrutiny of a small cluster of principles — while highly formal and abstracted from any attempt to root them in a horizon of meaning — constitutes a (restricted) form of interpretation of meaning, especially when this scrutiny is viewed against the background of the political experiences from which the principles indirectly arise. This would be true, for example, of *Principles of Biomedical Ethics* by Tom L. Beauchamp and James F. Childress, 3rd ed. (New York: Oxford University Press, 1989).

ethical theories — but with a free and open look at the meaning of the experience of human life and destiny.[23]

What do we mean by the experience whose meaning is to be interpreted? It is not merely an objectively described empirical entity, for experience (etymologically, to survive or live through a crisis) includes the notion of the agent's perception.[24] Experience is not fully separable from meaning, because human experience is written on the horizon of meaning. To use a phenomenological term, we are dealing with an antepredicative experience, in which the original nucleus of what moral consciousness perceives is preserved in the unity it has prior to the distinctions brought about by faculties of reason, will, sentiment, and so on.

What do we mean by the meaning of such a reality? To apprehend the meaning of something is to understand and make a judgment about an experience (or about one sphere of the entire world of experience), so as to appreciate its significance and know how to live with and respond to its significance.

The search for meaning is no novel recommendation in today's scholarly world. There is a blossoming of the search for meaning in human studies generally: for example, in women's studies (the meaning of women's lives, roles, perceptions, ways of reasoning); in ethnographic and anthropological studies (e.g., describing and translating cultural systems of meaning); in philosophical schools of thought (e.g., examining, through hermeneutical epistemology, the meaning of handicap, illness, wellness); and in theology (e.g., examining the significance of the experience of grace, of the lived ecclesial community, etc.).

The objection is sometimes raised, at least implicitly, that questions of meaning are only of secondary importance in contemporary ethics, particularly in clinical medicine, where the primary reality with which

23. See Warren Thomas Reich, "Experiential Ethics as a Foundation for Dialogue Between Health Communication and Health-Care Ethics," *Journal of Applied Communication Research* 16 (1988): 16-28.

24. See, for instance, the important comments made by Gadamer on the concept of experience and the meaning of hermeneutic experience: Hans-Georg Gadamer, *Truth and Method,* trans. Joel Weinsheimer and Donald G. Marshall, rev. ed. (New York: Continuum Publishing Co., 1994), 265-380. For an application of this concept in ethics, see Dietmar Mieth, *Moral und Erfahrung: Beiträge zur theologisch-ethischen Hermeneutik* (Freiburg i. Br.: Herder, 1977).

we must deal is the making of tough decisions in a concrete clinical, technical, and moral context. In this perspective, "gazing into the meaning of things" is an exercise not meriting much of our attention.

It does indeed make good sense to put meaning in a secondary place and give primacy, instead, to one's immediate reality, in situations in which infants and afflicted adults must be concerned with living or surviving, with learning (or relearning) how to speak, walk, hear, and eat — and how to differentiate and combine these experiences in ever larger syntheses. But as mastery and use of language develop in the child or its broader use returns to the afflicted, we come to live, "not in the world of immediate experience, but in a far vaster world that is . . . mediated through meaning."[25]

The task and challenge of incorporating the search for the meaning of moral experience in (bio)ethics is best understood by examining elements of moral epistemology that reach out for or actually incorporate the interpretation of meaning. I will briefly consider those elements individually and include examples of bioethical thought that have already taken a move in this direction, as well as examples that provide an agenda for the task that lies ahead.

1. Moral Decision-Making

When the larger world of wellness, suffering, being struck with affliction, being sick, dying, parenting, nursing, and so on is not mediated in the decision-making process of clinical ethics — when, instead, clinical ethics mechanically relies on an algorithmic approach to solve its moral problems by utilizing a step-by-step procedure involving the standard concepts and the standard sources (advance directives, patient consent forms, values inventory, proxy consent forms, etc.) — clinical ethics ultimately creates an obstacle to good habits of moral reasoning and hinders the flourishing of bioethics, even if, ironically, such concepts and procedures produce the "right" answer for the question that was asked.

It must be acknowledged, of course, that an ethic which, in principle, aspires to the interpretation of all reality — or all relevant reality — is certainly never a fully closed ethic, nor will it ever offer the

25. Lonergan, "Dimensions of Meaning," 253; see also 252.

full certitude that some versions of classical ethics claimed. Nevertheless, an ethic based on the search for meaning is a manageable and useful approach to ethics, for it engages first one carrier or embodiment of meaning and then another, in dialogue — whether those carriers be found in language, symbols, history, art, anthropology, a person's incarnate meaning (her actual story, her actual way of life), story, theories, principles, and so on. Some promising inquiries into "carriers" that in fact shape contemporary clinical ethics include works dealing with value-laden narratives of health-related experiences,[26] the uses of power by clinicians,[27] and, in general, the link between the theory and the practice of medical ethics in the clinical experience itself.[28]

Moral decisions are made in dialogue regarding meaning. The agent discovers metaphors to enlighten an entire range of behaviors, and images, models, and patterns to guide actions. Sometimes the actions are simply those of facing the ordeal of illness, of persisting faithfully to be present to the other, or of enacting a (secular) ritual — say, in transplant surgery or in companying the dying — as a means of preserving or creating moral meaning and "legitimizing" a continued reflection on moral, personal, professional, and spiritual meaning.[29]

Some authors argue that the dominant mode of judging and deciding is not formal logical argument but discernment, a sort of prudential or practical reasoning which deals with a complex set of

26. See Arthur Kleinman, *The Illness Narratives: Suffering, Healing, and the Human Condition* (New York: Basic Books, 1988); Kathryn Montgomery Hunter, *Doctors' Stories: The Narrative Structure of Medical Knowledge* (Princeton, N.J.: Princeton University Press, 1991); and Rita Charon, "Narrative Contributions to Medical Ethics: Recognition, Formulation, Interpretation, and Validation in the Practice of the Ethicist," in *A Matter of Principles? Ferment in U.S. Bioethics,* ed. Edwin R. DuBose, Ronald P. Hamel, and Laurence J. O'Connell (Valley Forge, Pa.: Trinity Press International, 1994), 260-83.

27. See Howard Brody, *The Healer's Power* (New Haven: Yale University Press, 1992).

28. See Richard M. Zaner, "Experience and Moral Life: A Phenomenological Approach to Bioethics," in *A Matter of Principles? Ferment in U.S. Bioethics,* ed. Edwin R. DuBose, Ronald P. Hamel, and Laurence J. O'Connell (Valley Forge, Pa.: Trinity Press International, 1994), 211-39; and Glenn C. Graber and David C. Thomasma, *Theory and Practice in Medical Ethics* (New York: Continuum Publishing Co., 1989).

29. See William F. May, *The Patient's Ordeal* (Bloomington: Indiana University Press, 1991), 1-14; and May, *The Physician's Covenant: Images of the Healer in Medical Ethics* (Philadelphia, Pa.: Westminster Press, 1983), 13-25.

epistemological factors through its elements of detecting, sensing, sifting, discriminating, comparing, connecting, and deciding.[30] This mode of moral decision-making is relevant to all settings, but in particular to the sort of context in which, for example, parents must accept or reject their own initiation into the art of parenting their severely handicapped infant. When parents decide whether and how to bond with and then care for their child, they may not follow moral rules and principles at all; they are more likely to experience the possibility of living out an image of parenting they discover in the context of a major transition from loss of the envisioned child to attachment to the one they received. That image carries moral normative force, in the sense that it makes possible a spirited rejection or spirited emulation of values and virtues.[31]

2. Care: The Root of Striving for Meaning

The primary root of the pursuit of meaning in moral knowledge is the metaphysical notion of care. Although the idea has a long history in mythology, philosophy, literature, and the practice of the care of souls, little systematic attention has been paid to the important function played by care or concern in the history of (moral) knowledge.[32] Writing within this tradition, Kierkegaard explained that consciousness — as distinct from disinterested reflection — is inherently *concerned* with both the knowing subject and what is known.[33] For Heidegger, the self *(Dasein)*

30. See James M. Gustafson, *Theology and Christian Ethics* (Philadelphia: United Church Press, 1974), and *Ethics from a Theocentric Perspective* (Chicago: University of Chicago Press, 1981). Ronald Carson has developed the notion of discernment in reference to bioethics in "Interpretive Bioethics: The Way of Discernment," *Theoretical Medicine* 11 (1990): 51-59.

31. See Warren Thomas Reich, "Caring for Life in the First of It: Moral Paradigms for Perinatal and Neonatal Ethics," *Seminars in Perinatology* 11, no. 3 (July 1987): 285.

32. The idea to which I refer is part of what I have called "the Cura tradition of care," which is a major element in the history of the idea of care. See my "Care: I. History of the Notion of Care," in *Encyclopedia of Bioethics,* ed. Warren Thomas Reich, rev. ed. (New York: Simon & Schuster-Macmillan, 1995), 319-31.

33. Kierkegaard, *Johannes Climacus; or, De Omnibus Dubitandum est; and A Sermon,* trans. Thomas Henry Croxall (Stanford, Calif.: Stanford University Press, 1958).

111

is care, in the sense that we understand and care about ourselves as beings-in-the-world because of our connectedness with being and action brought about by care. Thus, at the root of what it means to be a self, it *matters* that we can act: we care about it.[34]

Charles Taylor carries forward, more systematically, the foundational importance of care as the driving force toward meaning in his definition of the human agent as person: "Agents are beings *for whom things matter,* who are subjects of significance." Because we are beings for whom things matter, we are, fundamentally, subjects who are open to matters of meaning or significance. Taylor continues: we evaluate self and life not essentially in light of fixed goals, but also and specifically in sensitivity to certain standards involved in peculiarly human goals.[35]

This theory of moral knowledge makes it not only relevant to, but even essential for, bioethics to consider such questions as these: How has a male-dominated culture shaped what it means to be a woman and the evaluation of her health needs? What does it mean for a woman to be a moral agent? What do women care about (say, regarding justice, abortion, caretaking roles, etc.)? Bioethics would be different and better if it were to acknowledge fully and integrate into its dialogue the voices of women in reply to these questions.[36] Similarly, the ethics of responding to aging and the elderly depends in great measure on discovering what it means to be an aged person.[37]

34. See Heidegger, *Being and Time,* new ed., trans. John Macquarrie and Edward Robinson (Oxford: Basil Blackwell, 1973).

35. Taylor, "The Concept of a Person," in *Human Agency and Language: Philosophical Papers,* vol. 1 (Cambridge: Cambridge University Press, 1985), 104-5. Alasdair MacIntyre, in his "Comments on Frankfurt" (*Synthese* 53 [1982]: 291-94), affirms the fundamental role of care for ethics: "The concept of *what we care about* assumes an importance in an area of our culture left vacant by the disappearance of a public theory of the good or of the hierarchy of goods. 'What is it important to care about?' replaces 'What goods ought we to desire?'" (291).

36. See Susan Sherwin, *No Longer Patient: Feminist Ethics and Health Care* (Philadelphia: Temple University Press, 1992); and Karen Lebacqz, "Feminism," in *Encyclopedia of Bioethics,* ed. Warren Thomas Reich, rev. ed. (New York: Simon & Schuster-Macmillan, 1995), 808-18.

37. An example of this sort of morally revealing inquiry is found in the work of Thomas Cole: *The Journey of Life: A Culture of Aging in America* (New York: Cambridge University Press, 1992); and *Voices and Visions: Toward a Critical Gerontology* (New York: Springer Publishing Co., 1993).

3. The Nature of Moral Truth

In contrast to the notion of truth as coherence, which has dominated our rationalist, argument-based approach to ethics, there is the often-overlooked notion of truth as manifestation. The latter notion of truth involves the power of disclosure and concealment on the part of the known object and the related experience of recognition on the part of the knowing subject. In every true manifestation, there is a dialogical interaction between the object's disclosure and concealment and the subject's recognition through interpretation. That interaction is conversation.[38]

This notion of truth makes evident the relevance of a variety of texts that are correlative to a number of modes of moral knowledge in ethics. For example, narratives — which are the primary way of articulating, organizing, and communicating the sense human beings make of the world — are the prime locus of truth-as-manifestation;[39] and moral dialogue with a story is almost guaranteed, for the story itself is interactive before the listener interacts with the story. Whether the narrative is a primordial Greco-Roman myth of healing, an autobiography of a victim of sexual abuse, or an African-American woman's poem about aging, it can richly manifest (and instruct us regarding what it conceals about) the elements of a situation to be addressed by another's response.[40]

The truth manifested in a variety of "texts," whether stories, shared experiences, or other forms, is usually initially perceived and interpreted, in conversation with the "text," as antepredicative or preconceptual knowledge, perhaps later to be more extensively formulated and eventually employed in argument.[41] Even as antepredi-

---

38. See David Tracy, *Plurality and Ambiguity: Hermenutics, Religion, Hope* (San Francisco: Harper & Row, 1987), 28-29.

39. See Stephen Crites, "The Narrative Quality of Experience," *Journal of the American Academy of Religion* 39 (1971): 291-311.

40. See Marian Gray Secundy, *Trials, Tribulations, and Celebrations: African-American Perspectives on Health, Illness, Aging, and Loss* (Yarmouth, Me.: Intercultural Press, 1992).

41. See David Burrell and Stanley Hauerwas, "From System to Story: An Alternative Pattern for Rationality in Ethics," in *Knowledge, Value, and Belief,* ed. H. Tristram Engelhardt Jr. and Daniel Callahan (Hastings-on-Hudson, N.Y.: Hastings Center, 1977), 111-52.

cative, however, moral knowledge is often operative and hence directly relevant to the moral discourse ingredient in ethics. Specifically, truths about the experiences of suffering, the harm done by neglect of suffering persons, and the good done by compassionate care of suffering persons — manifested through literature, psychology, autobiographical accounts, moral-anthropological models, and so on — can, through interpretive dialogue, give rise to a new (or renewed) ethic of responding to suffering.[42]

4. Moral Agency and Intentionality

The two previous sections, on care and the nature of moral truth, have both presumed the turn of ethics to the subject of morality, to the moral agent. An ethic that begins with meaning takes seriously the moral agent, who typically cares about the moral life, who stands, so to speak, behind moral language, but who has been lost behind the veil of anonymity created by a universal and impersonal ethic.[43]

The moral self or moral subject is recaptured, in part, by Husserl's notion of intentionality.[44] Since ethics involves the study of all experiences and/or clusters of experiences that have a bearing on the moral life, ethics must (as Husserl claimed phenomenology must) involve the study of the objects of experiences, because experiences are *intentional*. Reference to an object is essential to experiences; and the reference of experiences to intentional objects consists of meaning. The content of this reference of moral experience to object is not accessible to the objectivity of an abstract rationality. It is "intuited" by thought that is synthetic, that takes feeling into account as part of rationality (as do Pascal's "reasons of the heart"), and that perceives the object in the unity of its meaning, as a world-for-me.

42. See, for example, Eric J. Cassell, *The Nature of Suffering and the Goals of Medicine* (New York: Oxford University Press, 1991); and Warren Thomas Reich, "Speaking of Suffering: A Moral Account of Compassion," *Soundings* 72 (1989): 83-108.

43. See Derek Parfit, *Reasons and Persons* (Oxford: Clarendon Press, 1984).

44. Husserl, *Ideas: General Introduction to Pure Phenomenology*, trans. W. R. Boyce Gibson (New York: Collier Books, 1962), 235-60.

114

This is the world of moral orientation and of moral character, for without a consideration of the role of moral character as the subject of evaluation, it would not be possible to assess the meaning of the intentionality of our moral experiences. In this sense, then, character and virtue form an essential part of the arsenal of the pursuit of moral meaning. Viewing the person as moral subject, Stanley Hauerwas argues for the primacy of character and narrative in philosophical and theological ethics. He regards character as the qualification of self-agency by the moral subject's beliefs and intentions.[45]

In light of these considerations, the role of moral character is an essential component in understanding, for example, the meaning of the experience of suffering due to blind overtreatment, the meaning of sexual molestation experienced as a shameful blow to one's self-identity, and the meaning of suffering due to an untimely terminal illness.[46] Furthermore, however, to the extent that virtue ethics becomes a set of fixed ideals that function more or less as a hierarchy of ordered goods, virtue and character lose their capacity to serve the pursuit of moral meaning, for in such a view they have abstracted from the moral agent as intentional subject, no matter how appealing they may be to the motivations of some agents.

Similarly, casuistry can be viewed as embodying the intentionality of a community — its orientation to meanings, values, and goods. It is the art of making use of a moral community's memory by bringing to bear on decision-making the ways in which paradigmatic cases embody the wisdom of the community in rhetorical language that is only minimally discursive. Viewed as such, it can be a major instrument in the task of the interpretation of moral experience. However, to the extent that casuistry is viewed simply as a set of skills for the practical application of moral principles, divorced from the moral community in which it obtains its meaning, it loses its capacity to serve as a tool to be used in the search for moral meaning.[47]

45. See Stanley Hauerwas, *A Community of Character: Toward a Constructive Christian Social Ethic* (Notre Dame: University of Notre Dame Press, 1981).

46. See May, *The Patient's Ordeal,* 1-15.

47. See Albert R. Jonsen and Stephen Toulmin, *The Abuse of Casuistry* (Berkeley: University of California Press, 1988). My explanation of the interpretive function of casuistry will not be found in the Jonsen-Toulmin work.

5. An Ethic of Moral Response

An approach to ethics that provides the impetus to unify the search for moral meaning and normative ethics is an approach that is symbolized by what can be regarded as the first question to be addressed to the task of ethical reflection: What is going on around me, and what would be a fitting response to what I (we) find addressed to me (us) in this moral world of mine (ours)? The question necessitates a repositioning of the stethoscope of ethics, from its position over a narrowly concentrated problem to a position where it can hear the totality of the significance of the experience or sphere of experience that is addressing the moral agent.

This approach to ethics is sometimes called an ethic of response. Both H. Richard Niebuhr[48] and Charles Taylor offer a moral philosophy of response; for example, Taylor describes a person as "a being who can be addressed, and who can reply." He calls the person a "respondent."[49] The response approach to moral analysis is forcefully elicited by Levinas's image of the face of the stranger.[50] I may ignore or respond to the stranger; and if I respond it may be with words, silence, or actions that meet his or her needs. I may reject or welcome the stranger's world into my world, but I will ineluctably be morally affected by the encounter. The greatest danger is that we, both as moral agents and as ethicists commenting on morality, will succumb to the temptation to domesticate all reality[51] by subsuming the totality of what the Other represents into our familiar categories of moral thought. What is needed in bioethics is a firm focusing on the meaning of the stranger-subject before us — whether the different-feeling woman or man, the differently endowed fetus or handicapped in-

48. Niebuhr, *The Responsible Self: An Essay in Christian Moral Philosophy* (New York: Harper & Row, 1963).

49. Taylor, "The Concept of a Person," in *Human Agency and Language: Philosophical Papers,* vol. 1 (Cambridge: Cambridge University Press, 1985), 97.

50. Emanuel Levinas, *Totality and Infinity: An Essay on Exteriority* (Pittsburgh: Duquesne University Press, 1969). Thomas Ogletree has situated the phenomenological thought of Levinas in the broader fields of philosophical and theological ethics in his work *Hospitality to the Stranger: Dimensions of Moral Understanding* (Philadelphia: Fortress Press, 1985).

51. David Tracy discusses this temptation in *Plurality and Ambiguity,* 51.

dividual, the different-skinned and different-speaking foreigner or native, or the hospital patient who has become a stranger by refusing to avoid the forbidden realm of death.

A response approach to moral interpretation and normative ethics is, I think, the most useful approach to developing a much-needed moral art of caring for the dying.[52] Principles of beneficence and the justification of withdrawal of treatment by appeal to "proportional" assessments in a calculus of benefits have only a limited reach in an ethics of dying; such moral language can conceal the larger question of moral response to the person who is attempting to have his or her own experience of dying. A response ethic in this area would focus on relational behaviors — on responses of companioning, communicating with, and showing compassion for the person who is in a unique situation of living through his or her dying days and hours.

6. The Role of Attention

Attention is the door through which we move to come into contact with moral experience and discover moral meaning; it is our window to the moral world. The word *attention* is taken from a Latin word whose radical meaning is "to stretch out to." One stretches out to a work of art or another human being by attending to it, her, or him; in this way the agent perceives and interprets the other.

Simone Weil, a philosopher who regarded attention as a pivotal idea, explained that it entails, above all, a negative effort. It consists of suspending our thought, leaving it detached, empty, ready to be penetrated by the (manifesting) object, ready to receive the being one is looking at, "just as he is, in all his truth."[53] It means waiting, seeking, being open to naked truth. For the realm of ethics, she rejects the adequacy of the Kantian notion of person. Attention to the person of the other is not at all helpful in discovering a useful moral norm;

52. James Bresnahan makes an appeal for a contemporary art of dying (not an art of *caring for* the dying such as I am advocating) in his "Death: Art of Dying: II. Contemporary Art of Dying," in the *Encyclopedia of Bioethics,* ed. Warren Thomas Reich, rev. ed. (New York: Simon & Schuster-Macmillan, 1995), 551-53.

53. Weil, *The Simone Weil Reader,* ed. George A. Panichas (New York: David McKay, 1977), 51.

rather, one must exercise positive moral attention to the individual as individual. Her notion of justice is one bred of a compassion elicited in the exercise of attention.

Attention is the master key to an ethic that this essay has advocated — one chiefly characterized by the search for the meaning of moral experience. It is also key to the major methodological elements of the "experiential" ethic I have described: interpretation, radical care, truth-as-manifestation, moral agency, intentionality, character, and response. Consequently, I believe that bioethics, in an era that would devote itself to a study of the meaning of moral experience, must examine in a more fully developed way the role of attention in moral epistemology, and what difference attention would make in clarifying and developing bioethics in a mode of moral response.

My final comment on attention is one directed to the purpose of this book, which is to examine the past and future involvement of theological and religious ethics in bioethics. Both the historical turn to the moral subject in ethics and the pressing need for a concerted turn to moral interpretation create a situation that breaks down the distinction between philosophical and theological ethics. While both of those disciplines make significant and separate contributions to special needs — for example, the needs to articulate the ethics of a particular religious community and to analyze particular moral concepts — the intellectual barrier dividing them breaks down in the arena of the public search for moral meaning.

In the contemporary cultural and intellectual setting that I have described, caring attention can be regarded as the starting point of, and the unifying factor for, all of ethics; and it is especially crucial for the development of a bioethics that would be responsive to our most pressing moral needs. Attention, however, is a contemplative sort of action; the contemplation it entails is contemplation of the moral significance of subjectivity. Both as regards its nature and its object, then, the attention required for interpretation is a spiritual act, in the sense that it entails regard for the very stuff of existence and its meaning, as well as regard for choices about one's existence — choices that imbue our world and our lives with the meaning that is symbolized by our basic moral language and responsiveness. Both philosophers and theologians have an important role to play in an ethic that is radically centered on a (secular) spiritual act.

The central role that attention to meaning should play in the future of bioethics convinces me that it is crucial that religious and theological scholars — for whom matters of meaning and interpretation are central to moral inquiry — participate more directly and more vigorously than they have in recent decades. Cooperation of this sort is needed for the development of a field of bioethics that is concerned with the meanings by which humans think out the possibilities of their own living and make choices among them.

Contexts for Medical Ethics and the Challenges for Religious Voices: Reports of the Working Groups

Working groups were an important part of the conference, providing an opportunity for conversation about the contributions of religious voices to medical ethics in the past and about an agenda for the future.

One set of working groups considered some of the contexts within which religious people work and struggle with questions of medical ethics: the academy, the medical center, the religious communities, and the public policy arena. Each of these contexts provides particular challenges to and opportunities for reflection about medical ethics by thoughtful religious people.

The working groups were asked to consider one of these contexts and to identify some contributions of theological reflection in the past, some possibilities for the future, some difficulties encountered by those who would work theologically there, and some suggestions to enhance theological reflection (and the contribution it can make) within that context.

1. The Academy[1]

Theology provided a framework and a tradition within which to think about health care, identifying moral concerns and formulating principled decisions. Even when members of the academy disagreed with the theological assumptions or with the particular conclusions, theological arguments about health care encouraged attention to the practical implications of fundamental accounts of human nature and destiny.

More recently theologians who have emphasized narrative have provided a less abstract approach to medical ethics. The focus on cases typical of medical ethics has continued, but the cases are sometimes described more fully and more richly than previously. Moreover, the agents involved in the cases are sometimes described amply enough to prompt consideration not only of the question "What should a rational and impartial (and self-interested) person do in a case like this one?" but also the question "What should this person, belonging to his or her particular communities and having her or his particular moral identity, do in this case?"

Departments of religious studies have, in comparison with departments of theology, typically less connection with particular religious traditions. This, combined with the pluralism of the university and the culture, has sometimes led to downplaying the distinctive features of a particular religious tradition. However, such departments have also been able to call attention to the inalienably religious character of decisions dealing with birth, suffering, death, and caring for the sick.

Those who would engage in theological reflection about health care within the academy face serious challenges. One challenge is the lack of theological literacy. Even those students and colleagues who belong to a particular religious community frequently have little competence in their own religious tradition and less in the language and tradition of other religious communities. At the very least those work-

---

1. The working group on the academy was chaired by Michael Allsopp and included Melvin J. Brandon, Coletta Dunn, Shimon Glick, J. Norman King, William H. Moorcroft, Donal P. O'Mathuna, Ann M. Parfitt, James C. Wagener, and Mary T. White.

ing in the academy must contribute to society by increasing theological literacy and thus enabling a better understanding and appreciation of the framework within which religious people have made decisions about the issues of health care in the past.

Other challenges, however, are provided by pluralism and the privatization of religion. The diversity of voices in the academy can be exciting and enriching, but too often the diversity simply mirrors the moral fragmentation of the culture. There are many voices, but there is little genuine dialogue. It is important for religious voices within the academy to resist the impulse of pluralism to treat religious convictions as purely private matters and as publicly irrelevant.

Such a challenge may be met in part by efforts to continue and to improve dialogue with other disciplines — and other interests — within the academy. Such an effort should preserve the autonomy of religious discourse while making religious models for discernment intelligible and, indeed, enriching them in the dialogue with other disciplines.

The working group suggested that theologians in the academy should play the role of a theological Socrates or an academic prophet, challenging all frameworks that undercut a life of integrity. They should challenge, for example, models for reflection about medical ethics that, for the sake of universality, alienate decision makers from the particular convictions, commitments, loyalties, and communities that give them both moral character and moral passion.

Finally, the group called for attention to limits: to the limits of medicine, to be sure, and to the limits of resources, but also to the limits of the academy. Many decisions will remain morally ambiguous, and the academy should not pretend to provide an escape from that ambiguity. Moreover, no academic course in bioethics is likely to be sufficient for the formation of character. Theologians in the academy can warn the academy against pride and remind it of the moral significance of other institutions and groups to serious moral discourse, character formation, and community.

2. The Medical Center[2]

Religious reflection and conversation were once more commonplace in the relation of patient and physician or nurse. Where caregivers and patients knew each other and their religious commitments, the ways in which religion motivated them and guided them entered into the conversation more easily. A number of things have conspired to make the clinical setting less hospitable to religious dialogue.

Among those things have been certain features of the medical center. The specialists and intensivists are typically strangers to the patient. The "technological atmosphere" can create a distance between the patient and the caregiver, and between both and those who would call attention to the presence of transcendent power. Moreover, the business of health care has encouraged the construal of the relationship of patient and caregiver as a commercial relationship of consumer and provider. The patient who enters a medical center is separated from most of what is familiar; it seems a different world, in which the traditions and rituals of the world left behind can seem out of place.

There are also features of our culture that have made theological reflection and religious dialogue more difficult in the medical center. The separation of church and state has been construed by some to prohibit attention to religious realities within any institution that receives state funds. There is the reality of pluralism both in the larger society and in the medical center itself — and a strategy for dealing with pluralism that makes religious convictions a private matter and "nobody else's business." And there is the increasing immersion in the secular.

There are, however, also features of theology that have alienated it from the medical center context. The focus of much theology on rational abstractions has sometimes seemed to discount the emotional

2. The working group on the medical center was chaired by Margaret McDonnell and included Armand H. Antonmaria, Dana L. Bainbridge, Elaine L. Cockerham, Maxine C. Glaz, Elizabeth A. Hawkins, Jean Ellen Herzegh, Dennis M. Maaske, Sandra C. Magie, Stephen L. Mann, Henry N. F. Minich, Robert W. Morton-Ranney, Alvin H. Moss, Jacek L. Mostwin, Maureen H. Muldoon, Robert M. Nelson, John F. Peppin, Lawrence A. Plutko, Robert D. Reece, Kent R. Roberts, C. Grant Story, Steven D. Thorney, Jan van Eys, Katherine van Eys, and George Webster.

life of both patients and caregivers. And the triumphalism of some theology has rendered it either threatening or irrelevant in situations of tragedy. The religious stories we tell seem sometimes distant from the human stories we are living or watching.

The working group saw no easy solution to the difficulties encountered by those who wanted to engage in theological work and religious dialogue within this context. Nevertheless, simply because there are many deeply religious people who undertake the practices of health care and want their health care profession to be coherent with their religious profession, and because there are many other religious people who give birth, get sick, suffer, and die, religious reflection and discourse can hardly be dismissed from the medical center.

The working group did identify some ways to enhance theological reflection within the medical center. It was suggested that theologians in this context have much to learn from their feminist colleagues, that an emphasis on care and relationships should at least supplement attention to freedom and autonomy. It was suggested that theologians might focus on the practices of religious people, that attention to rituals of piety might at least supplement attention to theological concepts. It was suggested that, if theologians want clinicians to take theology seriously, they should listen to doctors and nurses speak of their triumphs and their tragedies, nurturing and sustaining the theological reflection that health care professionals themselves are driven to undertake. It was suggested that those who wish to encourage religious dialogue in the medical center must resist the impulse to think that they can dispense "God" to patients like so many aspirin; let them rather start with the assurance that God is already present and continue by being attentive to God's mysterious presence.

The working group cited David Smith's proposal of "paired concepts" as useful to the medical center and pushed it in the direction of not only pressing for coherence between certain secular ethical concepts and theological concepts but also pressing for coherence between certain professional and/or patient behaviors and certain religious practices. By discerning the sacred in the secular, it might be possible to nurture and sustain a sense of calling among caregivers and a sense of integrity among patients, and it might also enrich the religious traditions within which we work.

3. The Religious Communities[3]

Religious communities have provided support for health care over the years in a variety of ways, building hospitals, providing volunteers, celebrating health care as a ministry, visiting the sick. Moreover, religious communities have provided the context for the moral formation of a number of individuals involved in health care ethics in a variety of other contexts. The churches have a very mixed record, however, with respect to providing a context for reflection about medical ethics.

Some religious groups seem to have so identified the culture of health care, especially compassion armed with technology, with the requirements of the gospel that they have sacrificed the capacity to be critical. The explanation may be found in the Baconian vision of Puritanism and of liberalism, but an uncritical identification was noted as a reality and as a problem. Some religious communities accept a dualism of body and soul and a division of labor apportioned by such a dualism; health care is assigned the task of caring for the body, while religious communities concentrate on the needs of the soul. Such communities regard health care as "none of their business" and properly left to the health care professionals; but at least occasionally they are forced to recognize the tension such a division of labor creates for patients, who are after all whole persons, and for caregivers, whether clinical or clerical. Some religious communities accept conventional health care, but not all of its practices. In these contexts the tendency is to construe medical ethics as a list of prohibitions. Some religious communities affirm alternative therapies, whether Christian Science or other spiritual healing, and among these groups there is sometimes a general suspicion of conventional health care. The religious communities provide not one context but several different contexts for theological reflection about the ethics of health care.

This lack of theological consensus is a problem not only across denominations but also within many denominations. Moreover, the

---

3. The working group on the church was chaired by Willard Krabill. Martha Kunau served as reporter. Other members of the group were Jan de Jong, Alice Gillen, Mary Hlas, Stephen C. Holmgren, Barbara T. Johnson, Robert T. Keller, George Luthringer, M. Therese Lysaught, Mary Schlachtenhaufen, David Smith, Kenneth Vaux, Allen Verhey, and Robert Weise.

task of the theologian is defined differently in different religious traditions.

Even so, the working group called on theologians and others to retrieve and articulate the tradition of particular communities of faith in ways that would enable them to engage in moral discourse and moral discernment as communities with a distinctive memory and hope. This will require attention to scripture and to the practices of prayer and the sacraments as they bear on the ordinary human events of giving birth, suffering, dying, and caring, and as they bear on the extraordinary powers of modern health care. It will require the diversity of gifts in communities of faith, and it will require attentive and humble listening not only to scripture and the tradition but also to each other, to those within the community who provide health care and to those who receive it. It will also require an ecumenical dialogue that does not attempt to eliminate differences by finding a lowest-common-denominator set of convictions, but that rather attempts always to renew the common life of a congregation by attention to the way strangers as well as saints read and live the story they remember and struggle to live.

Theological reflection in these contexts will issue often in a priestly word of support for those who suffer and for those who care for them, sometimes in a prophetic word challenging an extravagant and idolatrous confidence in technology, sometimes in a sage word about life in a mortal body and in community. Such words will best serve communities of faith and their dialogue and discernment when they are spoken out of and for the religious communities themselves.

There will be occasions for religious communities or their representatives to speak to "the world," and it will be appropriate, of course, to be as persuasive as possible in speaking with those outside the community, but the working group urged religious communities and voices to distinguish themselves from interest groups and their lobbyists, to speak in public out of their convictions and commitments.

The working group made a number of practical suggestions to enhance theological reflection in these contexts. Support groups for health care professionals and for patients should be formed in congregations, attending to God and to all else, including their care and their pain, as related to God. Adult religious education should involve health care professionals and patients who are willing to talk and to

126

listen about discipleship within their roles. The voices of women should be heard in the churches on these issues. Pastors need continuing education opportunities in medical technology and in moral theology. Books and articles on religious integrity and health care need to be written for congregational use.

4. Public Policy[4]

Historically, religious values have shaped or influenced the culture and public policy within the culture. Certainly the social gospel, exemplified by Walter Rauschenbusch, had an impact on American culture and policy. So, too, Reinhold Niebuhr's critical realism influenced policy makers. As David Smith observed in his paper at the conference, religion was an important influence in the education and moral formation of many important figures. Within health care, it must be observed that respect for the "religious values" of patients has been an important part of patient care, reinforced and upheld by case law and stipulated by the requirements of JCAHO (Joint Commission on Accreditation of Healthcare Organizations). Religious leaders made significant contributions to the President's Commission studies.

Rauschenbusch's ambition of "Christianizing" the social order may now seem pretentious, but more modest ambitions of preserving some little good, avoiding some great evil, or simply being a "leaven" are important enough to warrant the best efforts of religious people in the public policy arena.

Many different suggestions were made by different members of the working group. One person invoked the work of Bellah and his colleagues to urge a renewal of "civil religion." The suggestion called for a religion of the polis to be kept distinct from the religions of particular communities of faith. Such a civil religion would be richer than "moral minimalism," but it would not warrant the enforcement

---

4. The working group on public policy was chaired by B. Andrew Lustig and included Alan B. Astrow, Warner Bailey, Amy Chambers Huber, Kathryn S. Jones, Lonnie D. Kliever, Timothy E. Madison, Thomas W. Nuckols, Grace M. Stuart, William Stubing, and Susan McPhail Wittjen.

of "moral maximalism." It would allow for diversity but would refuse to privatize religion.

Another suggestion invoked "levels of argument" with respect to public policy and urged a distinction between the warrants for public policy, which ought to be kept free from expressly religious language, and the backing for those warrants, which could involve religious convictions and theological concepts. The religious backing provided does — and should — frame and shape the warrants, but without altogether eliminating the capacity of common warrants to guide policy formation. It was observed that the suggestion is similar to proposals of "middle axioms."

A reaction to the first two proposals suggested that both "civil religion" and "middle axioms" functioned at a far higher level of generality than the level at which most public policy discussion is — properly — conducted. Religious people involved in these discussions need something more than general principles and something other than abstract theological concepts. They need, it was suggested, to be in conversation not only with other policy makers but also with a community of faith that tells a story that is not immediately applicable to policy formation but that does form the virtue and the vision of the one engaged in the "art of the possible."

Another suggestion followed up on this remark, observing that the most important role for the religious communities with respect to public policy may be the shaping of conscience and character, not only among those directly involved in policy formation but among citizens. The cultivation of virtue is a necessary precondition to a higher level of public debate and concern.

There was a concern that religious communities must recover a prophetic voice in the public policy context, even if we would not want the prophets to write policy.

The discussion kept returning in various ways to the question of whether a public morality was necessarily minimalist. The group was not willing to forgo what it took to be the necessary attempt to find common ground, and it was willing to acknowledge that such common ground was not as rich and fertile as the language of faith, but it hoped that the presence of religious voices might serve to "elevate" the lowest common denominator.

The group identified a variety of difficulties encountered by those who would work with theological integrity in this context. A certain construal of the "doctrine" of the separation of church and state, unhistorically and often polemically, is used to preclude religious voices from the public square. Pluralism in the larger culture has led to regard for "unqualified" reason and science as the only legitimate authorities and to regarding religion as a "private" matter. Pluralism in the churches has, on the one hand, made it difficult to build a consensus within the churches about public policy issues and, on the other, made it important for more moderate perspectives to distinguish themselves from extreme and intolerant religious voices. There is a perception that the media are suspicious and hostile toward religious voices and ignorant of religious traditions. There is the difficulty of "translating" religious perspectives into a "public language." And when policy issues are viewed as straightforwardly "religious" issues, compromise becomes more difficult.

The group recommended serious study of public policy issues by religious communities, continuing education opportunities sponsored by denominations and ecumenical organizations, continued appropriate presence in the development of legislation, including public statements, position papers, and testimony at public hearings.

At the close of its session one of the members of the working group reminded the rest that theological reflection about public policy is important but not sufficient for at least two reasons. First, policy formation itself is only one of the arenas in which religious people are called to be active publicly and, perhaps, not the most significant of those arenas. Second, reflection must be joined to action, to public words and deeds that bear witness (even if indirectly) to their convictions.

Some Issues and the
Future of Theological Reflection:
Reports of the Working Groups

A second set of working groups focused on some issues and the possibilities and challenges of theological reflection concerning them. The issues were abortion, genetics, assisted suicide, and access to health care. Each group focused on one issue, attempting to summarize and assess the specifically religious contributions to the discussion of this issue in the past and to identify some elements of an agenda for future theological reflection about this topic. Having heard most of the major addresses at the conference, the working groups frequently identified themes from the presentations that they regarded as particularly instructive or provocative for future consideration of their particular issue.

1. Abortion[1]

The working group noted that in "the Abrahamic religious traditions" there have been significant restrictions on abortion. These traditions

1. The chairperson of the working group on abortion was Stephen Holmgren; the group also included Warner Bailey, Dana Bainbridge, Shimon Glick, Mary Hlas, Alvin H. Moss, Kent R. Roberts, Mary Schlachtenhaufen, William Stubing, and Mary T. White.

provided the background assumptions with respect to abortion for centuries. Among those assumptions is a view of the preeminent value of human life as compared with animal life, a view illustrated in the creation accounts, in the view of human beings as spirit bearing, and in a variety of texts, like Psalm 8, for example.

Talmudic texts on the sanctity of life were noted, as was the emphasis there on the requirement of procreation. Also noted were the Christian doctrines of the incarnation and the resurrection and their implications for the concept of the *imago Dei*. A generally consistent emphasis on the sanctity of human life has been the consequence of these teachings and doctrines, even where there have been different accounts given of the conditions sufficient to overcome the presumption in favor of life in instances of abortion.

Furthermore, the working group contrasted the early Christian preference for a *substantial-historical* concept of the human person (evident in Christology), emphasizing the givenness of vocation as the core of one's identity, with the more *qualitative*-based concept of human personhood in classical thought, a concept linked with the possession of certain attributes. The *substantial-historical* concept can be connected with such texts as God's words to the prophet Jeremiah in the "call" passage (Jer. 1:5), words like those also found in Psalm 139:13-16.

The working group suggested that an agenda for theological reflection about abortion should surely include continuing reflection on these themes and background assumptions. It also identified the vocation of parenthood, of being a mother or a father, the concept of "family," and the "necessity" or "desirability" of offspring as items that belong on the agenda for theological reflection. The working group suggested the importance of theological reflection concerning abortion used as a means of contraception or for convenience, and it suggested that such reflection be joined to the issues of a "contraceptive mentality" and the place of technology within such a mentality. The working group urged attention to the theme of stewardship and to its bearing on both the use of personal and family resources (the issue of family planning) and the use of global resources (the issue of the familial appropriation of those resources). The themes of autonomy and control and self-determination will remain on the agenda. Finally, the working group suggested that a fresh consideration of the neglected doctrine of providence as an alternative to accounts of our lives governed by fate or by chance could contribute to a fresh consideration of abortion.

The working group observed that the agenda will and should be formed, at least in part, by future medical and scientific developments relevant to abortion. It noted, for example, the continuing development of RU-486 pills, the technology that makes "viability" earlier and earlier, the emergence of fetal medicine, and the identification of the fetus in medical textbooks as "a patient."

Members of the working group commented on the theme of "alien dignity" as fruitful for future consideration of abortion in communities of faith. Some called attention to Karen Lebacqz's compelling account of the legacy of Helmut Thielicke as a resource for emphasizing a human dignity that characterizes a being *irrespective* of any particular qualities or traits. Others called attention to her emphasis that the implications of "alien dignity" include the protecting and equalizing of those with such dignity. And others called attention to her account of the importance of relationality as instructive for a reconsideration of the moral status of the fetus.

Warren Reich's paper was also seen by members of this group as offering an important methodological shift to theological consideration of this bioethical issue as well as many others. Specifically, his account of "attention" and "care" seemed to some members of the group to be instructive not just with respect to the acts themselves but also with respect to the ones those acts intend, the one *to whom* we attend, the one *for whom* we care. It was suggested that we learn "who is the neighbor" not so much by exegetical inference or conceptual analysis but by attending to another as neighbor, by caring for another as neighbor.

The group pointed out the theme of "marginalization" in more than one of the presentations, and it noted the apparent ineffectiveness of the theological traditions with respect to abortion in public controversy. Here it found James Gustafson's heuristic models for discerning various approaches in religious ethics to be of help in understanding how religious views may be shaped and communicated. It also noted that, with the development of science and technology, for example, with the development of RU-486, abortion may in the future be no longer quite so *public* a decision. It may no longer require clinics or involve the courts in such an obvious way. Even so, abortion itself, by whatever means, will remain an issue of concern for religious ethics; it may be important now to consider how different approaches are appropriate to different audiences and not to allow public policy disputes to monopolize theological reflection about abortion.

2. Genetics[2]

Genetics has been an issue since before the beginnings of bioethics, and religion has been involved in the moral conversation about genetics from the beginning. The working group noted, for example, the debate between Paul Ramsey and Joseph Fletcher concerning genetic control at the beginnings of bioethics. Their debate about genetics touched on issues of human freedom, embodiment, the control and mastery of nature by technology, the responsibilities of parents and the limits on those responsibilities, the appropriate goals for genetic interventions and the appropriate means to achieve those goals, and eschatology. Those issues remain important to the debate about genetics, and they continue to invite theological reflection.

The working group began by noting some different contexts for theological reflection about genetics: the public policy (and scientific policy) arena, the clinical context, and religious communities. The role of theological and religious reflection will vary according to the context.

Within the public policy arena, the working group said, theologians should be participants, if for no other reason than that a genuinely pluralist society does not silence distinctive voices. Moreover, policy with respect to genetics will affect the lives of religious persons. They and the people who study and articulate their religious traditions should be given a hearing. The major role within the public policy arena was identified as providing categories to cor-

---

2. The chairperson for the working group on genetics was M. Therese Lysaught; other members included Alan B. Astrow, Jan de Jong, Elizabeth A. Hawkins, Barbara T. Johnson, Kathryn S. Jones, Sandra C. Magie, Stephen L. Mann, Ann M. Parfitt, James C. Peterson, Robert Morton-Ranney, Maureen H. Muldoon, Rebecca D. Pentz, Grace M. Stuart, Walter L. Wagener, and Robert Weise.

rect, confirm, and augment the public discussion. These categories would include the image of God, created cocreators, original sin, finitude, and others. The categories are of limited public usefulness because they belong within substantive and specific traditions, but their limited usefulness does not make them of no use to the public discussion. Moreover, the group acknowledged that these categories can sometimes cut against each other; for example, the categories of cocreators and finitude can sometimes support different dispositions toward genetic research and technological innovations. Even so, theological reflection can contribute to the public policy arena not by providing a formula, but by encouraging a process open to critical reflection about the quasi-theological assumptions hidden in secular arguments.

Religion plays a role in the relationship of practitioner and patient. Too little reflection, in the view of the group, has been done concerning this arena. Genetics counselors, for example, are not pastoral counselors, but neither are the persons with whom they deal objective utility calculators; they are sometimes religious people who have traditions and communities that provide certain resources for dealing with tragedy and for discerning appropriate judgments with respect to certain risks. Moreover, genetics counselors, by their commitment to nondirective counseling and by regarding as an open question an option that a person's religious tradition has closed, may willy-nilly be present at a moment of spiritual crisis. The working group suggested that reflection about this arena belongs on the agenda of both geneticists and religious leaders, and it encouraged conversations between genetics counselors and pastoral counselors.

With respect to religious communities as an arena for theological reflection, the working group noted that such communities are where many people live who will be affected by genetics. More people who face personal decisions about what to do with genetic information and technology are members of particular religious communities than of, say, the society for the advancement of impartial rationality. In this arena substantive and tradition-specific theological reflection is surely called for. The educational programs of congregations should include both information about genetics and also reflection about the relevant resources of the particular tradition, for example, the liturgies for marriage and baptism.

The communities of faith and their theologians ought to exercise sometimes a prophetic role and sometimes a pastoral role, according to the working group. The prophetic role should be undertaken with respect to eugenic proposals; with respect to genetic discrimination, whether explicit or not; with respect to the notion of "perfectibility," even when it occurs under cover of the notion of "genetic health"; with respect to the tendency toward genetic reductionism (for example, in the oversimplified one-to-one correlation between genes and traits); with respect to the notion of "ideal" or "normal" human beings; with respect to regarding children as products; with respect to the pretensions of medicine when proposing technical solutions to what are nontechnological problems; and with regard to funding priorities relative to health (that is, funding for genetics research in comparison to funding for the public health needs of nutrition, sanitation, and treatment of basic infectious diseases).

The working group also challenged communities of faith to play a pastoral role with respect to these issues, to be a place where "burdens" are shared and thereby lessened, to be a place where we train to love the imperfect, to be a place where suffering prompts a compassion armed not only with technological artifice but with wisdom about life in a mortal body and in community and with piety.

Looking back on their discussion, the working group observed that the remarks of Karen Lebacqz concerning alien dignity and about relationality had been pulled into the discussion and that the analysis by Stephen Lammers of the arenas for theological reflection had helped shape the discussion.

3. Assisted Suicide[3]

The working group on assisted suicide began its discussion by marking terminological and definitional distinctions between passive and active

3. The chairperson of the working group on assisted suicide was Lonnie Kliever; other members included Armand Antonmaria, Jean Ellen Herzegh, Amy Chambers Huber, Robert T. Keller, J. Norman King, Willard Krabill, Martha A. Kunau, George Luthringer, Timothy E. Madison, Margaret McDonnell, Henry N. F. Minich, Jacek L. Mostwin, Robert M. Nelson, Thomas W. Nuckols, Donal P. O'Mathuna, John F. Peppin, David L. Smith, C. Grant Story, and George Webster.

euthanasia and physician-assisted suicide and physician-administered euthanasia. Passive euthanasia *allows* the patient to die from the underlying disease; active euthanasia *causes* the patient to die by medical intervention. In the latter case, in physician-assisted suicide, the physician provides the medical means of suicide; in physician-administered euthanasia, the physician applies the medical means of death. While some thinkers reject the distinctions between passive and active and between physician-assisted suicide and physician-administered euthanasia, the working group accepted these as morally significant distinctions. The group decided to focus its discussion on physician-assisted suicide.

Opening discussion revealed strong, though not unanimous, opposition to physician-assisted suicide in the group. It was observed that the moral, legal, and professional strictures against physician-assisted suicide have been supported by the Jewish and Christian traditions. Traditional theological emphases on the sanctity of life, the value of suffering, the promise of eternal life and the threat of eternal damnation, and the limitations on human freedom have raised powerful barriers against self-chosen death. Suicide has been widely seen as a sin against self, others, and God. Even in the case of human extremity, suicide violates our own nature, breaks faith with the human community, and usurps the sovereignty of God. As such, suicide is frequently regarded as inherently self-centered and sinful within Jewish and Christian traditions.

The group observed that the implication of these religious traditions has not usually been taken to be that human life must be preserved "at all costs." It noted that, within these traditions, withholding or withdrawing treatment at the request of the terminally ill patient is usually theologically and morally licit. The Catholic tradition has long allowed a distinction between extraordinary and ordinary means and has recognized the principle of double effect. These provide ways of sanctioning the termination of treatment; extraordinary means (means that are hard to obtain or excessively burdensome to a patient, or that provide an insufficient chance of success) are not morally obligatory; and palliative care that is intended to relieve suffering and that has the effect of hastening death is not culpable according to the principle of double effect, provided that the intention is to do good and the bad consequence, even if foreseen, is not a means to achieve the good consequence. Neither of these principles, however, can be stretched to support active euthanasia as long as suicide is categorically forbidden.

Having noted these emphases in their religious traditions and the moral, legal, and professional strictures against physician-assisted suicide that these emphases support, the group raised the question of why public interest in and approval of physician-assisted suicide has risen so dramatically in recent years. Several reasons were suggested: the American commitment to radical autonomy, fear of the process of dying, mistrust of the medical profession, the insistence on a *right* to die. While most early efforts to legalize physician-assisted suicide failed at the ballot box, this matter remains a live issue in the public perception, despite the remedies offered through advance directives and durable power-of-attorney assignments.

Some members of the group would support assisted suicide in extreme cases of unrelieved suffering; some thought a physician who had a long and personal relationship with the patient could provide the means for that release from suffering. However, those of the group who took such a view were not in favor of *legalizing* assisted suicide, because legalization would open the door to abuses.

The group identified some theological and religious concerns that might provide some support for physician-assisted suicide. The requirement to relieve suffering was noted, and the implications considered for cases of voluntary death in the face of debilitating disease with the long-term expectation of suffering and degradation. The possibility that death might be chosen as an act of sacrificial love for others was noted, and the categorical separation of martyrdom and suicide was questioned.

In its conversation the working group recognized a number of questions that belong on the agenda of those who would reflect theologically about this issue. What do individuals in situations of extremity owe the community? Do we have the right to require all to die a heroic death? Does human freedom encompass the freedom, in Thielicke's words, to give our souls back to God by our own hands? Does God require that we die a "natural death"? Does God demand that we suffer? What is the meaning of suffering? What does a community owe those who are suffering? Are there limits to the responsibility to relieve suffering? Is there a distinction between relieving suffering and eliminating suffering? Is the sanctity of life relevant to a life reduced to organic functioning, or is it related to the life lived in responsive and responsible relationships? All of these questions raise the fundamental question: can there be a self-chosen death that is an affirmation of the sanctity and solidarity of human life?

The working group urged that the agenda should include not only theological reflection about these questions but also the search for common ground for affirming the sanctity of life in the public square. It called attention to David Smith's "paired concepts" proposal and to James Gustafson's model for a dialectical relation of religious reflection with other forms of moral reflection as methodologically useful suggestions, and it noted that Karen Lebacqz and Warren Reich offered important theological and anthropological "starting points" for such a search.

It also urged a reexamination of the meaning of suffering in religious traditions and in human experience, particularly the suffering unto death. It observed that Warren Reich addressed this question most directly by turning our attention to questions of meaning and care.

4. Access to Health Care[4]

Care for the sick poor has been part of the historic mission of religious hospitals, certain religious orders, and medical missionary work. Such care was not regarded as charity or as a matter of right, but as faithfulness to an identity and a vocation formed in religious community. The "Good Samaritan" responded to human need, and the conclusion of the story invites those who hear it to "go and do likewise." Such stories, and the stories of Jesus as healer and preacher of good news to the poor, have formed and continue to form Christian character and community. These were among the items mentioned when the working group on access to health care identified some contributions

4. The chairperson for the working group on access to health care was Allen Verhey; other members included Melvin J. Brandon, Elaine Cockerham, Coletta Dunn, Alice Gillen, Maxine C. Glaz, Dennis M. Maaske, Willaim H. Moorcroft, Lawrence A. Plutko, Robert D. Reece, Steve D. Thorney, Jan van Eys, Katherine van Eys, and Susan McPhail Wittjen.

of Jewish and Christian religious traditions to the concern for providing access to quality health care.

There have also been some contributions to a recognition of the scarcity of resources and to the need to distribute scarce resources fairly. The notion of stewardship has played a role in theological reflection about resources and would reward reexamination. It was also mentioned that attention to a life after death by God's grace and power made care for the sick an appropriate task but a limited responsibility. The triumph over death was understood finally as a divine victory, not as a technological achievement. And note was also taken of the ways in which the principle of love and the principle of justice have interacted in the culture and as standards for decision with respect to access to health care. An assortment of "classic" pieces on this interaction were mentioned.

The agenda for theological reflection about health care reform must include, according to the working group, a challenge to the mythology of medical technology. Specifically, theologians have a public obligation to challenge the assumption that medicine provides transcendence over the human limitations of mortality, finitude, and vulnerability to suffering. Unless extravagant (and idolatrous) expectations can be set aside, it will be difficult to limit medical expenditures. Moreover, the Protestant theologians in the group acknowledged some special responsibility for challenging the "Baconian" assumptions that knowledge is power over nature and leads almost inevitably to human flourishing, since the "Baconian Puritans" had played a role in fostering such views in the culture. Some members of the group suggested that a parallel claim needed to be made with respect to extravagant expectations of the marketplace as a mechanism not only to encourage innovation but also to distribute goods fairly. The claim was not that religious narratives could be "translated" into public policy proposals for health care reform but that public policy frequently (and in this case) is accompanied by stories and assumptions, some of which need public correction.

The working group suggested that the agenda should include reflection about compassion and justice, not simply as impartial principles, but as tradition-formed virtues. Compassion, for example, as a response to suffering is concretely formed by our culture's confidence in technology as a remedy for suffering. If that confidence is challenged, compassion may be formed again and trained to respond to suffering in nontechnical ways. And the "justice" formed by a story of self-interested and rational strangers forced to create a contract for their life together (as, e.g., in John Rawls's "original position") will be a little more tightfisted than the "justice" formed by a story of the rescue of a bunch of slaves from Egypt. However, the working group also suggested that virtues besides compassion and justice belong on the agenda for theological reflection about access to health care and health care reform, including, for example, truthfulness, humility, gratitude, and fidelity.

The agenda should include efforts by religious communities to get their own stories straight. The group noted, for example, that the practice of prayer is sometimes undertaken as a "spiritual technology," whether as an alternative or as a supplement to conventional medical technology, and that sometimes the expectation of a miracle is given as a reason to continue what is regarded as "futile" treatment. It was also noted, in this context, that the religious traditions have not only convictions but liturgies that are relevant to "sharing," that it can be asked, as Paul did with respect to a Corinthian celebration of the Lord's Supper where some had plenty and others had none, whether we eat and drink judgment to ourselves if we fail to share.

The working group foresaw some version of "two-track care," and it was prepared to accept such a system if it assured everyone access to decent health care. It was suspicious, however, that "two-track care" would deteriorate into a two-class system. It urged involvement in policy development to protect against such a consequence; it urged the character formation of doctors and nurses so that they would be advocates for their patients and especially for their medically indigent patients, both with administrators and with policy makers; and it urged the religious communities to continue programs of health care ministry to meet some of the needs of some of the poor in their parishes and neighborhoods.

There was much in the presentations of the conferences that would reward attention by those who would reflect theologically about the issues surrounding access to health care. James Gustafson's point about the importance of various descriptions of the same reality was underscored by more than one member of the group. The relevance of an economic analysis, a medical analysis, a philosophical analysis, and a policy analysis was admitted by everyone, and no one claimed that a theological analysis could be substituted for any of them. The contribution of theological reflection may be particularly related to the narratives that form character and to the prophetic words that beat against injustice, but they are also related (and for some members of the group, particularly related) to philosophical ethical analysis or to public policy analysis. Those who saw their role in relation to philosophical analysis found David H. Smith's "paired concepts" proposal helpful, especially but not exclusively with respect to love and justice and covenant and contract.

Some members of the group commented on Warren Reich's attention to "meaning" as important to expanding the horizons with respect to the reasons for assuring access to health care. Health care is important publicly not simply because of the value of life or the entitlements of rights, but because it is one of the ways the community signals care for one another in the midst of suffering and tragedy.

Karen Lebacqz's account of "alien dignity" as a protective notion was appreciated. The group acknowledged scarcity as one reality of the health care discussion; Karen Lebacqz helped us to see the sanctity of each of those in need as loved by God. When scarcity and sanctity meet, it may not be possible (or morally required) to do everything for everyone, but the failure to do all we can for one person who is the object of God's uncalculating love is not therefore "good"; the importance of an "uneasy conscience" in situations where evils gather and cannot all be avoided is an important legacy from Thielicke for health care reform and an important protection against two-track care slipping into a two-class system.

MEDITATION
Is the Last Word "Darkness"?

ALLEN VERHEY

Call to Worship:

(from Psalm 99)

> LEADER: The Lord reigns; let the peoples tremble!
> God sits enthroned; let the earth quake!
> The Lord is great in Zion, exalted over all the peoples.
> Let them praise your great and awesome name.

> ASSEMBLY: Holy is God!

> LEADER: Mighty Ruler, lover of justice,
> you have established equity;
> you have executed justice and righteousness in Jacob.
> Extol the Lord our God; worship at his footstool.

> ASSEMBLY: Holy is God!

A Thanksgiving for the Saints:

(from Revelation 7:9-17 and Matthew 5:3-16)

> LEADER: There was a great multitude that no one could count,
> from every nation, from all tribes and peoples and lan-
> guages, standing before the throne and before the Lamb,

robed in white, with palm branches in their hands. They cried out in a loud voice, saying:

ASSEMBLY: Salvation belongs to our God who is seated on the throne, and to the Lamb!

LEADER: And all the angels stood around the throne and around the elders and the four living creatures, and they fell on their faces before the throne and worshiped God, singing:

ASSEMBLY: Amen! Blessing and glory and wisdom and thanksgiving and honor and power and might be to our God forever and ever! Amen!

LEADER: Then one of the elders addressed me, saying:

ASSEMBLY: The one who is seated on the throne will shelter them. They will hunger no more, and thirst no more. The Lamb at the center of the throne will be their shepherd. And God will wipe away every tear from their eyes.

LEADER: Let us give thanks to God for all the saints.
Blessed are the poor in spirit.

ASSEMBLY: For all those humble and simple people who have been eager to help and ready to serve those who are sick and those who care for them, we give thanks.

(think of one such person, and give thanks)

LEADER: Blessed are those who mourn.

ASSEMBLY: For all those who shared the hurt of one who suffered and helped to bear the burden of pain, we give thanks.

(think of one such person, and give thanks)

LEADER: Blessed are the meek.

ASSEMBLY: For all those who attended carefully and respectfully to the needs of the dying, innocent of any concern for their own glory and power, we give thanks.

(think of one such person, and give thanks)

LEADER: Blessed are those who hunger and thirst for righteousness.

ASSEMBLY: For all those who longed for justice for the sick poor and worked for it, we give thanks.

(think of one such person, and give thanks)

LEADER: Blessed are the merciful.

ASSEMBLY: For all those who have been quick to kindness and slow to judgment, we give thanks.

(think of one such person, and give thanks)

LEADER: Blessed are the pure in heart.

ASSEMBLY: For all those whose devotion to the truth has made them suspicious of half-truths and self-deception, ready to endure the truth and eager both to learn and to do it, we give thanks.

(think of one such person, and give thanks)

LEADER: Blessed are the peacemakers.

ASSEMBLY: For all those who by word or deed bring some small token of the shalom God promises, we give thanks.

(think of one such person, and give thanks)

LEADER: For the grace that was given to all of these, and for the grace with which they touched the lives of others, we give thanks.

You are the salt of the earth; but if salt has lost its taste, how shall its saltiness be restored? You are the light of the world. A city set on a hill cannot be hid. Nor does one light a lamp and put it under a bushel, but on a stand, and it gives light to all in the house. Let your light so shine before others that they may see your good works and give glory to your Father in heaven.

Scripture:

Hear the word of God in the lament of the psalmist.

Psalm 88: O Lord, my God, I call for help by day;
I cry out in the night before thee.

Is the Last Word "Darkness"?

Let my prayer come before thee,
    incline thy ear to my cry!
For my soul is full of troubles,
    and my life draws near to Sheol.
I am reckoned among those who go down to the Pit;
    I am a man who has no strength,
like one forsaken among the dead,
    like the slain that lie in the grave,
like those whom thou dost remember no more,
    for they are cut off from thy hand.
Thou hast put me in the depths of the Pit,
    in the regions dark and deep.
Thy wrath lies heavy upon me,
    and thou dost overwhelm me with all thy waves.
Thou hast caused my companions to shun me;
    thou hast made me a thing of horror to them.
I am shut in so that I cannot escape;
    my eye grows dim through sorrow.
Every day I call upon thee, O Lord;
    I spread out my hands to thee.
Dost thou work wonders for the dead?
    Do the shades rise up to praise thee?
Is thy steadfast love declared in the grave,
    or thy faithfulness in Abaddon?
Are thy wonders known in the darkness,
    or thy saving help in the land of forgetfulness?
But I, O Lord, cry to thee;
    in the morning my prayer comes before thee.
O Lord, why dost thou cast me off?
    Why dost thou hide thy face from me?
Afflicted and close to death from my youth up,
    I suffer thy terrors; I am helpless.
Thy wrath has swept over me;
    thy dread assaults destroy me.
They surround me like a flood all day long;
    they close in upon me together.
Thou hast caused lover and friend to shun me;
    my companions are in darkness.

Psalm 88 is the saddest of the laments that are found in the Psalms. Most of the laments end on a note of praise — but not Psalm 88. Most of the laments finally express and delight in the faith of Israel — but not Psalm 88. All of the laments cry out to God — like Psalm 88: "O Lord, my God." And all of them describe the sad situation of the psalmist — like Psalm 88: "My soul is full of troubles. My life draws near to Sheol. I have no strength."

Many of the laments remind God that the dead are dead and cannot praise him — like Psalm 88: "Do the dead rise up to praise you? Is your steadfast love declared in the grave?" All of the laments close with a vow to give praise to God or with the expression of the certainty that God will hear their prayer and rescue them. All of them — except Psalm 88.

Psalm 88 is the saddest of the laments. It has no final word of praise or assurance or hope. The last word of Psalm 88, the last word for this psalmist, is "darkness." "Darkness" is the last word.

Now, I do not want to be too hard on this psalmist. One gets the impression that people apparently had been hard enough on him already. But is the last word "darkness"?

We can understand the psalm, I think. Indeed, we can sympathize with this pathetic man — and it might do no harm to start there. After all, even the dullest heart among us knows what the man is saying. He is sick — and he has been sick since he was a boy. "From my youth up," he says, "I have been afflicted and close to death."

Some have supposed the man a leper or palsied, but whatever the proper diagnosis, he would have been regarded as under the power of death, and he now suffers his way toward death.

At first, of course, all his family and friends rallied around him in his tragedy. His family tended to his needs, and his friends visited him. But the years have taken his parents, and made his affliction uninteresting to his friends. Now his friends seem to him to shun him and his loved ones to despise him. Now he lies there accompanied only by pain and death — and he cries, half to God, half to the air: "God! Listen to me! I am sick and tired! I am forsaken and forlorn! I am helpless and hopeless! My companions shun me. My friends despise me. My loved ones forsake me. And you hide your face from me. Listen to me!" And the last word is "darkness."

We can be sympathetic, I say, and we should be — for while we may not share his disease or his pain, none of us is altogether a stranger to his suffering, to his loneliness and sadness. Still, can we accept this? May we own this sad song as our song in our suffering, in our loneliness and sadness? Is the last word "darkness"?

Now, there is something in me and perhaps there is something in you that wants to shout angrily down the centuries back to this sad man, "Don't be so pitiful and self-pitying! Quit your complaining and trust God!"

The anger in that cry, our impatience with complaining, with the self-obsessed whimperings that "nobody loves me," is understandable enough, I suppose, but it is hardly commendable for all that. The man is in genuine torment — and our anger will not help.

Set aside our anger, then, our impatience with complainers; there is something else in us, something we think of as the grace of God in us, that makes us want to bridge the centuries with a word of hope. "It's not true," we long to tell the man. "The last word is not darkness, but light. The last word is not death, but life. Remember that the other psalms and other psalmists end with confidence in God and with the certainty of a hearing."

Jews might remind him that the last word of the Hebrew canon is Cyrus's word to the people in exile, a word in fulfillment of promise, a word of liberation for the people who dwelt in darkness, an invitation to go up to Jerusalem to worship God. "Let him go up," he said.

And Christians might remind him that the last word of the Christian canon is a cry of hope, a petition for the coming of God's good future — speedily and soon. "Maranatha." "O Lord, come."

But both would insist that the last word is life, not death; light, not darkness. And they would be right, of course. If God is God and faithful to God's promises, then the last word cannot be darkness. If God is God and faithful to God's promises, then we may not despair. Let it be said and said clearly then — against every temptation to despair — that Psalm 88 is wrong, that the last word is not darkness.

But what shall we make of Psalm 88, then? Should we rip it from our Bibles and discard it as insufficiently hopeful? This sad song is not just the pathetic cry of a miserable old man, it is God's word to us and for us.

I will grant that this psalm is not God's last word. The word of

147

God's grace and peace, the word of God's mercy and justice, shalom — that is and will be God's last word.

Psalm 88 is not God's last word, but it is God's word. And unless we hear it clearly and face it honestly, we may cheapen and domesticate the message of hope and joy, the announcement that God's word is not — and will not be — darkness, but light and life.

Psalm 88 *alone* would tempt us to despair. But *without* Psalm 88 — without this reminder of human suffering and of the silence of God, without this testimony of the anguish and helplessness even of one who surely is to be counted among God's people, without such a word from God — we would be tempted to triumphalism, to the sort of spiritual enthusiasm that supposes that righteousness and faith provide a charm against sickness and sadness, or that prayer works like magic to end our suffering and grief or to deliver our flourishing — or at least an answer to our questions.

Without Psalm 88, without this reminder of human suffering, without such a word from God, we would be tempted not only to spiritual triumphalism but to medical triumphalism, to the sort of technological enthusiasm that supposes that some new piece of medical wizardry will finally rescue the human condition from its vulnerability to death and suffering.

It is a temptation with us and on us whenever we would deny or ignore the sadness of this world, whenever we think our religion or our technology gives cheap and easy remedies for its sufferings, whenever we suppose that our faith eliminates its tragedy, or resolves its ambiguity into simple and clear answers. The temptation is with us and on us whenever popular preaching promises to dispense peace of mind, security, wealth, success, fame, and happiness — not to mention health and the remedy for suffering — in palatable doses of possibility thinking and calls that the hope of faith.

The prophets who suffered for the sake of God's word in a world like this one knew better. The martyrs who died for the sake of God's cause in such a world knew better. And that Jew I call Christ taught his disciples not how to avoid suffering but how to share it, how to endure it for the sake of others and for the cause of God in a world like this one.

The last word is not darkness, but the darkness sometimes deepens, and the enemy forces of pain and tears and death and oppression have not yet laid down their arms and admitted defeat. Triumphalism is not an option for Jews or for Christians, not until Messiah comes at any rate, or — as Christians say — comes again.

People die still, and die sometimes premature and horrible deaths. People suffer still, and suffer from causes sometimes too many to name and sometimes too powerful to fight. People ask still, and there is silence still. People seek still, and still do not find. People bloody their fists with their knocking, and there is yet no answer.

It is a sad world — and Psalm 88 is an antidote against any Pollyanna triumphalism, even when Pollyanna is a believer. So, Psalm 88 is a word from God, after all. And there are at least two lessons in this lament, one for those who suffer and hurt, and one for those called to minister to them.

First, the lesson for those who would minister to the suffering. It is this: Don't pretend that faith or medicine gives us easy answers. We may not simply say, "We will pray for you and it will be all right." We may not simply promise a technological rescue from mortality or from suffering. We may not simply say to the sick poor, "Do a little possibility thinking, and it will be all right."

Two things go along with this. First, we must *work* on the hard answers. We must work on the institutions that bend human life toward justice or toward violence, toward health or toward destruction. We must work on the real possibilities and on the real obstructions to human flourishing in community — even as people lie sick or dying.

And second, we must recognize that even with piety and with work, the darkness will sometimes deepen. We take courage for the work not in the pretense that we are messiah but in the confidence that God's last word remains to be spoken.

Sometimes the work we must do is simple presence, simply to be there, present to the one who hurts — silent ourselves perhaps with the voiceless sharing of another's pain, or if we open our mouths, ready not to attempt an easy answer but to share the lament, ready to make it ours as well in a com-plaintive cry.

That is a lesson for medicine's ministry to the suffering, too — a revisioning of medicine from attention to pathology to attentiveness to patients, a reform of medicine that arms compassion not only with artifice but with wisdom, including the wisdom of life in a mortal body in a world which is not yet — still, sadly, not yet — God's good future. Such a medicine can be present to the suffering and dying without panic, without the anxious effort to substitute for an absent God.

But there is another lesson in Psalm 88, a lesson for those who suffer and lament and cry out to God — and against God — in anger and in anguish.

It is simply this: They may. They may.

The community of faith accepted the words of this psalmist as God's own word. Cautions against despair are still in order. One may not indulge in self-pity, but one may be honest with God — and with a community that would take seriously the presence of lament, and such a lament, in its canon.

One may cry out, "The darkness deepens. Lord, with me abide."

Prayer:

ASSEMBLY: Good Lord, abide with us.
When the darkness deepens, good Lord, abide with us.
In the shadow of death, good Lord, abide.
In the gloom of suffering, good Lord, abide.
When we cannot see the good, in ambiguity and
uncertainty, good Lord, abide with us.
Help of the helpless, abide with us,
and help us to be present to others,
to give help to the helpless by your grace. Amen.

Contributors

James M. Gustafson is Henry R. Luce Professor of Humanities and Comparative Studies at Emory University. He is the author of many works, including the two-volume *Ethics from a Theocentric Perspective*.

Stanley Hauerwas is Professor of Theological Ethics at the Divinity School, Duke University. His many works include *Suffering Presence: Theological Reflections on Medicine, the Mentally Handicapped, and the Church* and *Naming the Silences: God, Medicine, and the Problem of Suffering*.

Stephen E. Lammers is Helen H. P. Manson Professor of Religion at Lafayette College and head of the department. He has edited, with Allen Verhey, *On Moral Medicine: Theological Perspectives in Medical Ethics* and *Theological Voices in Medical Ethics*.

Karen Lebacqz is Professor of Christian Ethics at the Pacific School of Religion, Graduate Theological Union, Berkeley, California. *Professional Ethics, Six Theories of Justice, Justice in an Unjust World*, and *Sex in the Parish* are among her many writings.

Warren Thomas Reich is Professor of Bioethics and Director of the Division of Health and Humanities at Georgetown University School of Medicine. A Senior Research Scholar at the Kennedy Institute at Georgetown University, he served as editor in chief of the *Encyclopedia of Bioethics* and of the revised edition of that widely acclaimed work.

CONTRIBUTORS

David H. Smith is Professor of Religious Studies and Director of the Poynter Center for the Study of Ethics and American Institutions at Indiana University. His many publications in moral theology and medical ethics include *Health and Medicine in the Anglican Tradition*.

Allen Verhey is the Evert J. and Hattie E. Blekkink Professor of Religion and Chairperson of the Religion Department at Hope College, Holland, Michigan. *Christian Faith, Health, and Medical Practice,* which he co-authored, and the works he edited with Stephen Lammers are among his contributions to the field.